NUCLEAR PHARMACY:

An Introduction to the Clinical Application of Radiopharmaceuticals

NUCLEAR PHARMACY:
An Introduction to the Clinical Application of Radiopharmaceuticals

Henry M. Chilton, Pharm.D.
Associate Professor
Department of Radiology
Division of Nuclear Medicine
Bowman Gray School of Medicine
Wake Forest University
Winston-Salem, North Carolina

Richard L. Witcofski, Ph.D.
Professor
Department of Radiology
Bowman Gray School of Medicine
Wake Forest University
Winston-Salem, North Carolina

Lea & Febiger   *Philadelphia   1986*

Lea & Febiger
600 Washington Square
Philadelphia, PA 19106-4198
U.S.A.
(215) 922-1330

Library of Congress Cataloging-in-Publication Data

Chilton, Henry M.
  Nuclear pharmacy.

  Includes bibliographies and index.
  1. Radiopharmaceuticals. I. Witcofski, Richard L.
II. Title. [DNLM: 1. Nuclear Medicine. 2. Pharmacy.
3. Radioisotopes. WN 440 C538n]
RM852.C48   1986   615.8′424   85-23910
ISBN 0-8121-1021-8

PRINTED IN THE UNITED STATES OF AMERICA

Print No.   4   3   2   1

TO OUR WIVES,

JUDY AND JANE,

AND OUR FAMILIES

Preface

The last decade has witnessed a remarkable increase in the variety of clinical nuclear medicine studies. The rapid advances in instruments have been more than matched by radiopharmaceutical development. The study of every organ system has been materially affected by the development of highly specific radiopharmaceuticals that generally provide more clinical information at a lower radiation burden than their earlier counterparts.

Although a source of considerable pride to the nuclear medicine community, this rapid growth in the variety of radiopharmaceuticals poses a formidable challenge to the student. In our experience there appears to be a need for an introductory text for students of nuclear pharmacy (including pharmacists, physicians, and technologists) covering the subject matter in depth sufficient to be of some permanent value, but presented in a clear and understandable manner. This book is our attempt to fill this need.

The organization of this text proceeds from basic principles to more practical aspects of clinical nuclear medicine. Because the book is intended to serve as an introductory text in nuclear pharmacy, the treatment of clinical applications is not exhaustive and presents only the major applications of each radiopharmaceutical. To facilitate study of clinical chapters, a general organization is followed: Principle of the study, indications, radiopharmaceutical data, methods, and special considerations/patient preparation.

The authors are indebted to their colleagues who helped in the preparation of this book. Nat Watson, Robert Cowan, Fred van Swearingen, David Williams, Larry Soderstrom, Steve Motsinger, and John Hawkins critically read portions of the manuscript. Much of the clarity that we have achieved in the text is due to their help. The obscurities that remain are ours.

We are also indebted to Douglas Maynard, our Department Chairman. His personal encouragement to each of us and the provision of an atmosphere that encourages academic achievement are greatly appreciated.

We also wish to express appreciation to Tom McDonald and the entire staff of the Nuclear Medicine Division of North Carolina Baptist Hospital for their assistance and encouragement during the preparation of this text.

Finally, we would be remiss if we did not express our indebtedness to Nina Haynes, Jan Rogers, and Carolyn Barber for their patient secretarial assistance, and to Teresa McAllister for her most valuable assistance in photography.

Winston-Salem, NC   Henry M. Chilton
Richard L. Witcofski

Contents

What Is Nuclear Pharmacy?

1.1 NUCLEAR MEDICINE

A discussion of nuclear pharmacy must begin with a description of nuclear medicine, since it is within this medical specialty that the radioactive products of nuclear pharmacy are used as diagnostic and therapeutic tools.

For practical purposes, nuclear medicine originated in the U.S. in 1946 when the Atomic Energy Commission (AEC) announced that by-product materials from nuclear reactors were available for shipment as medicinals. Clinical applications of these materials soon followed, and the concept of nuclear medicine was born. Originally, nuclear medicine was a minor subspecialty usually practiced within the fields of radiology, pathology, and internal medicine. Recognition that nuclear medicine procedures were reliable and possessed high benefit-to-risk ratios soon led to the creation of the specialty practice of nuclear medicine.

In the years that have followed, extensive developments in radionuclide production technology have increased substantially both the number and types of radioactive materials useful in a variety of clinical situations. The availability of high quality radiation imaging devices at reasonable prices has made it possible to institute nuclear medicine services at most hospitals.

The recognition of the value of nuclear medicine caused the Joint Commission for Accreditation of Hospitals (JCAH) in 1971 to require that all hospitals with more than 150 beds provide nuclear medicine services in order to be accredited. It has recently been estimated that more than 50% of the nation's hospitals offer nuclear medicine services and that these facilities account for more than 12 million patient doses of radioactive materials annually. Today in the U.S., over 10,000 physicians at approximately 3500 sites are licensed to use radioactive materials routinely.

1.2 RADIOPHARMACEUTICALS

The radioactive materials used in medicine were initially called "radiotracers" since they were most commonly radioactive forms (radioisotopes) of stable elements (such as iodine and calcium), or radioactive analogues of stable elements, and were used to follow (or trace) the biodistribution of the stable elements. Over the years, the term "radiotracer" gave way to "radioactive pharmaceutical," which has more recently been shortened to *radiopharmaceutical*.

A radiopharmaceutical is defined as a radioactive drug. Although this definition implies that a druglike (i.e., therapeutic) effect is associated with their use, radiopharmaceuticals usually do not elicit any pharmacologic response and are used primarily for diagnostic purposes (more than 90% of all radiopharmaceuticals are used as diagnostic agents).

For simplicity, radiopharmaceuticals can be thought of as having two components: (1) *a radioactive atom*, which gives off radia-

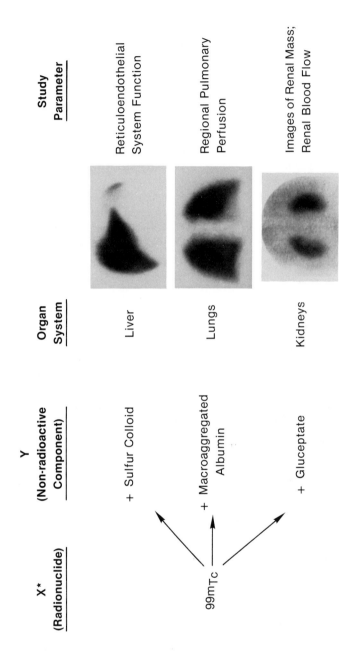

Fig. 1–1. The radionuclide Tc-99m can be used to "label" several nonradioactive substances to allow studies of different organ systems.

tions necessary for detection, and (2) *a non-radioactive component*, which provides the radiopharmaceutical with its distinctive chemical or physical properties.

The chemical form of the radiopharmaceutical may be simple, such as a salt, in which the nonradioactive component is an ion (such as Na^+ or Cl^-) and has little effect upon the biological behavior of the radiopharmaceutical. Most of the early radiotracer-type agents were salt-type agents whose biological distribution depended on the elemental properties of the radionuclide (e.g., radioactive iodine for thyroid imaging). More often, however, the nonradioactive component of most radiopharmaceuticals is complex (e.g., a chelate or

particulate) and provides characteristic properties that greatly influence tissue distribution.

In practice, a single radionuclide may be used to image several different organs simply by complexing the radionuclide onto a variety of tissue-specific compounds. For example, while the radionuclide Tc-99m (as ^{99m}Tc-sodium pertechnetate) is useful for performing thyroid gland imaging, Tc-99m can also be used for liver imaging when complexed to sulfur colloid, or for lung imaging when prepared as ^{99m}Tc-macroaggregated albumin (Fig. 1–1).

Images depicting radiopharmaceutical localization (called "biodistribution") are known as *scintiphotos* (Fig. 1–2) and are ob-

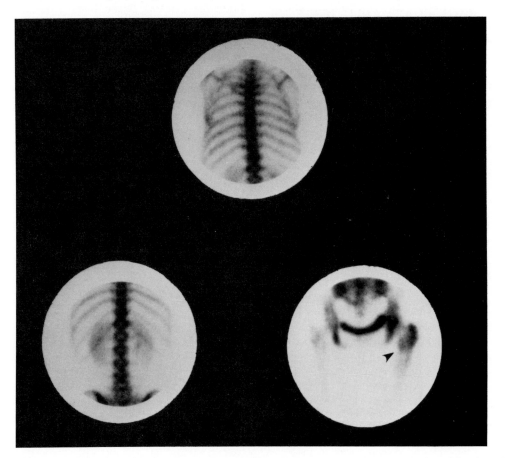

Fig. 1–2. Scintiphotos of a patient injected with Tc-99m medronate, a radiopharmaceutical used for skeletal imaging. This radiopharmaceutical concentrates in bone in relation to bone metabolic activity. For example, compared to the radiopharmaceutical uptake in normal bone, relatively greater uptake of this radiopharmaceutical occurs in areas of trauma and tumor as a result of the higher rate of bone turnover (*arrow*).

Table 1–1. Agencies that regulate the use and distribution of radiopharmaceuticals.

Food and Drug Administration (FDA)
Nuclear Regulatory Commission (NRC)
  (formerly Atomic Energy Commission)
State and Local Radiation Protection Agencies
  (in agreement states)*
Department of Transportation (DOT)
State Boards of Pharmacy
Environmental Protection Agencies
  (federal and state)

*In several states, NRC functions are performed by state agencies.

tained with a radiation detection device called a scintillation camera.

1.3 RADIOPHARMACEUTICALS VS. TRADITIONAL (NONRADIOACTIVE) PHARMACEUTICALS

Traditional (nonradioactive) pharmaceuticals are usually supplied by the commercial manufacturer in ready-to-use form, while approximately 85% of all radiopharmaceuticals must be compounded (or prepared) daily. Usually, this process is straightforward—often all that is required is the addition of a radionuclide (such as ^{99m}Tc) to a vial (or "kit") that contains the compound to be labeled (Fig. 1–3) and any other components necessary for radiolabeling.

Since most radiopharmaceuticals are administered parenterally, aseptic techniques must be used during preparation. As with traditional pharmaceuticals, the well known tests for sterility and apyrogenicity required by the Food and Drug Administration (FDA) are also required of radiopharmaceuticals. These tests are usually performed by the radiopharmaceutical manufacturer. Special types of radiopharmaceutical quality control tests may be necessary to ensure that optimal radiolabeling has occurred. These tests are usually performed by the user soon after the radio-

I. Manufacturer's Responsibilities
   1. Prepare compound to be radiolabeled *and* other necessary reagents (i.e., the "kit")
   2. Adjust pH, sterilize, lyophilize
II. On-Site Responsibilities
   1. Add desired radionuclide in specified quantity

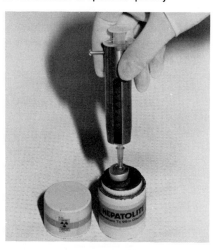

   2. Perform necessary quality control tests
   3. Dispense in prescribed activity for desired time

Fig. 1–3. Steps involved in on-site preparation of most radiopharmaceuticals.

pharmaceutical has been prepared and prior to its actual clinical use.*

Because radiopharmaceuticals are classified by the FDA as drug products, they are subject to regulations that govern the distribution and use of legend-type ("prescription") drugs. Further, since these special drugs are radioactive, federal and state agencies other than the FDA often regulate various areas of radiopharmaceutical use and distribution (including transportation and disposal). Some of these agencies are listed in Table 1–1.

Since December 17, 1984, the FDA has required that nuclear pharmacies comply with all applicable provisions of the Federal Food, Drug, and Cosmetic Act. The FDA has made available a document setting forth the criteria for determining at what point a nuclear pharmacy (or similar establishment) must register as a drug establishment. A description of these guidelines is found in Chapter 18.

The Nuclear Regulatory Commission (NRC) is the primary federal agency involved in regulating the handling, use, and disposal of radiopharmaceuticals. This agency also establishes and verifies training and experience requirements for the physicians who use these agents, the pharmacy personnel who dispense them, and the technologists who often administer them.

1.4   NUCLEAR PHARMACY

The concept of nuclear pharmacy was first described in 1960 by Captain William H. Briner while at the National Institutes of Health in Bethesda, Maryland. Briner's description of nuclear pharmacy services included the assistance of pharmacists in the procurement, preparation, quality control, and dispensing of radiopharmaceuticals. Originally, many of these tasks had been performed by technologists or others acting under physician authorization as part of the daily operation of nuclear medicine departments. With specialization, however, the logical participation of pharmacists in nuclear medicine evolved.

Types of Nuclear Pharmacies

Basically, the two kinds of nuclear pharmacy services existing today depend largely on the site and the types of nuclear pharmacy services provided.

Institutional nuclear pharmacy services are usually operated from either hospitals or large medical centers and may be staffed by hospital pharmacy personnel or more frequently, by pharmacists who are full-time personnel of the nuclear medicine department. In the past, many of these nuclear pharmacies have offered their services to nearby, smaller nuclear medicine departments but more recently, these services have become the basis of commercial enterprises.

Commercial centralized nuclear pharmacies, which are usually not affiliated with either universities or medical centers, provide their services to subscriber hospitals. Although these hospitals are usually nearby, they can be a drive of several hours from the nuclear pharmacy. Centralized nuclear pharmacies usually prepare and dispense radiopharmaceuticals as unit doses that are delivered to subscriber hospitals by nuclear pharmacy personnel.

Nuclear Pharmacists' Activities

In many ways, a nuclear pharmacy is like a traditional pharmacy; that is, prescriptions are filled, orders are processed, and records of inventory and dispensing are maintained. It is the unique radioactive nature of the radiopharmaceuticals used in the nuclear pharmacy that requires special

---

*Ideally, during radiopharmaceutical preparation almost all of the radionuclide should label the desired compound. Otherwise the subsequent clinical use of the material may result in poor-quality scintiphotos as well as the risk of potentially higher patient radiation exposure.

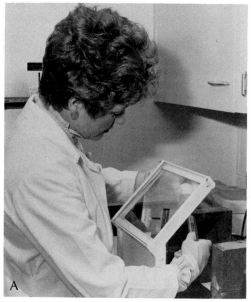

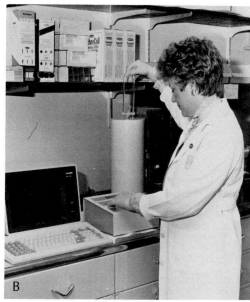

Fig. 1–4. (A) Preparation of a radiopharmaceutical dose using a lead barrier shield with a leaded viewing glass. (B) Prior to patient administration, doses should be assayed for radioactivity in a radionuclide dose calibrator. (C) Lead syringe holders are used to transport doses of radiopharmaceuticals to patients.

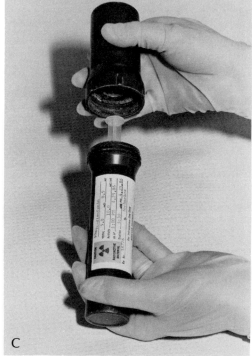

consideration in their handling, preparation, and dispensing.

Prescriptions for radiopharmaceuticals may be transmitted by telephone or issued as a part of the patient's nuclear medicine study request. Regardless, requests should include the following information:

1. the patient's name
2. the names of the requested nuclear medicine study and radiopharmaceutical
3. the amount of radioactivity to be administered
4. the time of administration (for short-lived radionuclides)
5. the name of the physician authorized to use the radiopharmaceutical

Occasionally, the pharmacist may review the patient's clinical history to verify the requested nuclear medicine study and the prescribed radiopharmaceutical. This is particularly important because many radiopharmaceuticals are appropriate for more than one clinical situation, and several agents may be useful in a given study. In these situations, the pharmacist should ascertain that the most desirable radiopharmaceutical has been prescribed.

Dispensing of Radiopharmaceuticals

Radiopharmaceuticals are prescribed according to units of radioactivity (either millicuries or microcuries) rather than as so many grams, milligrams or milliliters.

The actual dispensing of the patient dose involves determining how much radiopharmaceutical (usually by volume) will be required to obtain the prescribed amount of radioactivity at a given time. Since radiopharmaceuticals are often prepared in advance of administration, calculations

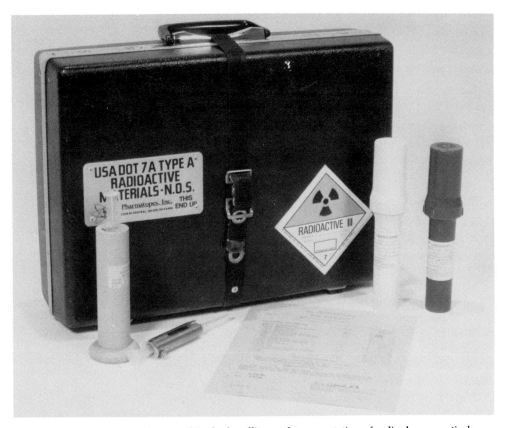

Fig. 1–5. Packaging and shielding used in the handling and transportation of radiopharmaceuticals.

Table 1–2. Selected nonradioactive drugs commonly used in nuclear medicine.

Drug	Use
Acid-citrate-dextrose solution (formula A)	Anticoagulant in cell-labeling procedures
Ascorbic acid	Reduction of excess chromate ion in procedures for red blood cell labeling with Cr-51 sodium chromate
Ceruletide	Stimulation of gallbladder emptying in hepatobiliary studies
Cimetidine	Inhibition of Tc-99m sodium pertechnetate washout from gastric mucosa in Meckel's diverticulum studies
Dexamethasone	Suppression of cortisol production in adrenal studies
Furosemide	Stimulation of urine flow in renal studies
Glucagon	Inhibition of Tc-99m sodium pertechnetate washout from gastric mucosa in Meckel's diverticulum studies
Heparin	Anticoagulant in procedures for red blood cell labeling with Tc-99m sodium pertechnetate
Hetastarch	Sedimenting agent in procedures for leukocyte labeling with In-111 oxine
Intrinsic factor	Adjunct in second-stage Schilling test
Laxatives	Bowel cleansing of intestinal radioactivity before Ga-67 gallium citrate imaging
Liothyronine	Suppression of thyroid function in thyroid studies
Lugol's solution	Inhibition of thyroidal uptake of radioiodide in studies with radioiodinated compounds
Potassium perchlorate	Inhibition of thyroidal uptake of radioiodide in thyroid studies; washout of nonorganified iodide from the thyroid gland in thyroid studies; inhibition of choroid plexus uptake of Tc-99m sodium pertechnetate in brain studies
Sincalide	Stimulation of gallbladder emptying in hepatobiliary studies
Thyrotropin	Stimulation of thyroid function in thyroid studies

should take into account corrections for loss of radioactivity by radioactive decay. Before dispensing, the amount of radioactivity in each radiopharmaceutical is assayed in a radionuclide dose calibrator (Fig. 1–4) to assure the accuracy of the dose.

Radiopharmaceuticals should always be handled and stored in lead-shielded containers (often called "pigs"). In addition, all patient doses must be properly labeled for the amount and type of radioactivity, and, if prepared for transportation, they must also be adequately packaged to protect against leakage and spillage (Fig. 1–5).

Because of special handling and storage requirements, prescribed doses of radiopharmaceuticals cannot be delivered to patients for self medication but must be administered by personnel trained and qualified to handle radioactive materials.

Finally, the residual radioactivity in used syringes and vials prohibits their immediate disposal as regular trash. These "contaminated" wastes may be returned to the nuclear pharmacy for proper storage and disposal.

Nuclear pharmacies also stock and dispense some nonradioactive drugs that may be given as pretreatments to either enhance or prevent the concentration of radiopharmaceuticals by certain organs. Several of these nonradioactive drugs, which include potassium perchlorate, Lugol's solution, thyrotropin, dexamethasone, and diuretics such as furosemide are shown in Table 1–2 along with their uses.

Pharmacists in Nuclear Medicine

Pharmacists have entered the specialized practice of nuclear pharmacy by several different routes. Pharmacists in the early 1960s were trained in nuclear medicine either by participating in short courses on the safe handling of radioactive materials or by receiving on-the-job training. Relatively few formal instructional programs in nuclear pharmacy were available. Today, several formal didactic and practical training programs exist for pharmacists. Upon completion of a bachelor of science degree in pharmacy, pharmacists may obtain additional training through nuclear pharmacy residency programs. Graduate courses and master's and doctoral programs in nuclear pharmacy are now offered by several universities.

A certification examination for pharmacists in nuclear pharmacy was established in 1982 by the American Pharmaceutical Association (APhA) through the Board of Pharmaceutical Specialties (BPS). This examination is offered annually to pharmacists with academic qualifications and on-the-job training experience in nuclear pharmacy. Additionally, the American Board of Science in Nuclear Medicine (ABSNM) offers an annual board examination (not limited to pharmacists) for persons who demonstrate competence in the combined areas of radiopharmaceutical and radiochemical sciences.

REFERENCES

1. Briner, WH: New dimensions for pharmacy. Hosp Top 43:79–90, 1965.
2. Briner, WH: Radiopharmacy: The emerging young specialty. Drug Intell Clin Pharm 2:8–13, 1968.
3. Distefano, RM, Hernandez, L: Clinical radiopharmacy. Drug Intell Clin Pharm 4:209–212, 1970.
4. Edwardine Sister Mary: The exciting challenge of radioactive isotopes. Hosp Progr 39:94–101, 1958.
5. Fincher, JH, Jones, FE: Current handling procedures of radiopharmaceuticals in U.S. hospitals. Am J Hosp Pharm 27:38–49, 1970.
6. Gnau, TR, Maynard, CD: Reducing the cost of nuclear medicine: sharing radiopharmaceuticals. Radiology 108:641–645, 1973.
7. Ponto, JA, Hladik, WB III: Common uses of nonradioactive drugs in nuclear medicine. Am J Hosp Pharm 41:1189–1193, 1984.
8. Quinn, JL III: The role of the hospital radiopharmacy. In Yearbook of Nuclear Medicine. Chicago, Yearbook Medical Publishers, 1970.
9. Report of the Joint Commission on the Accreditation of Hospitals, 1984, pp. 84–105.
10. Robinson, RG: Nuclear pharmacies: Organization, administration, and the regulatory agencies. Appl Radiology 6:162–166, 1977.
11. Subramanian, G: The role of the radiochemist in nuclear medicine. Semin Nucl Med 4:219–228, 1974.
12. Thrall, JH, Swanson, DP: Diagnostic Interventions in Nuclear Medicine. Chicago, Yearbook Medical Publishers, 1985.
13. Wolf, W: Radiopharmacy: A new profession. Hospitals 47:65–68, 1973.

Radioactivity

This chapter deals with the radioactive portion of radiopharmaceuticals, that component which makes them distinct from ordinary pharmaceuticals and permits their detection or measurement by radiation detection devices. In nuclear pharmacy, an understanding of the radioactive processes and the changes that occur in radioactive atoms is essential, since the modes by which radioactive atoms become stable determine the types of radiations emitted and hence their clinical utility. Also, since radioactive decay constantly decreases the amount of radioactivity present, technologists, pharmacists, and physicians must understand basic decay calculations in order to correct for loss of radioactivity with time.

2.1   HISTORICAL BACKGROUND

In 1896, Becquerel observed that uranium ore was capable of blackening photographic plates and ionizing gases. Two years later, the Curies called this phenomenon "radioactivity" and demonstrated its occurrence in other naturally occurring elements (radium, polonium, and thorium). In 1910, Rutherford and Soddy explained *radioactivity* as a process that transforms atoms of an unstable element into a stable element through the emisison of radiation. In the early 1930s, several important developments occurred: the production of artificial radioactivity was reported by Curie and Joliet, the neutron and deuteron were discovered, and the cyclotron was in-vented. To date more than 1500 artificial radionuclides have been produced by devices such as cyclotrons, nuclear reactors, and particle accelerators.

2.2   STABLE VS UNSTABLE ATOMS

Some atoms are stable while others are unstable and radioactive. Why? The reason seems to involve the number of protons and neutrons in the atom. In stable atoms that are small and less complex, the number of protons and neutrons is essentially equal. For example, stable phosphorus has 15 protons and 16 neutrons. As atoms become larger, however, relatively more neutrons must be present for stability (stable iodine, for instance, has 53 protons and 74 neutrons).

If the proton to neutron ratio does not lie within a narrow range of stability, the atomic nucleus is unstable and tends to change to a more stable proton to neutron ratio in a random, atom-by-atom fashion. The change from one nuclear form to another is called "radioactive transformation" or, more commonly, *radioactive decay* and involves the emission of energy. In the radioactive process, the number of radioactive atoms actually decreases with time, and the activity is therefore said to decay. The amount of time required for any given number of atoms of a radionuclide to reach half its original activity is called the physical half-life and varies among most radionuclides.

2.3 NUCLEAR NOMENCLATURE

The nucleus of an atom is characterized by the number of protons and neutrons it contains. For any element (X), the number of protons determines the *atomic number* (Z), while the total number of protons and neutrons is the *mass number* (A) of the nucleus. The format for representing these numbers is:

$$_Z^A X$$

When any two atoms have the same number of protons but a different number of neutrons, they are said to be *isotopes* of that element. Such atoms have the same elemental properties since they have the same number of protons. For example, there are three isotopes of hydrogen: hydrogen ($_1^1H$), deuterium ($_1^2H$), and tritium ($_1^3H$). Two of these, hydrogen and deuterium, are stable, while tritium is radioactive.

The term "radioisotope" should be used only in connection with radioactive forms of a particular element. For example, it would be incorrect to say "tritium is a radioisotope," but it would be correct to say "tritium is a radioisotope of hydrogen." When considering an atomic form with a specific number of protons and neutrons, the term *nuclide* is preferred. Thus, a specific radioactive atom would be called a *radionuclide*, and it would be correct to say "tritium is a radionuclide."

2.4 RADIOACTIVE DECAY SCHEMES

The modes of radioactive decay can be conveniently represented as line drawings, called decay schemes, which provide a detailed description of how an unstable atom decays. The changes in energy that occur during radioactive decay are represented by transitions from higher to lower energy levels and can be thought of as the rungs on a ladder (Fig. 2–1).

Transitions that involve only a change in energy are drawn as arrows straight down (Fig. 2–2). Those involving a reduction in the number of protons are indicated as an arrow slanting down to the left, while those that involve an increase in the proton number are shown by an arrow slanting to the right.

2.5 RADIOCTIVE DECAY

Types of Radiations

Alpha Particles. In the decay of a heavy, naturally occurring radioactive atom, alpha particles (α) are emitted from the nucleus. Alpha particles are composed of two protons and two neutrons and are the least penetrating type of radiation (absorbed or stopped by a few centimeters of air or a thin piece of paper).

Beta Particles. These high-speed electrons originate in the nucleus and can be either negative (β^-) or positive (β^+). In air they travel several meters, and in tissue, up to a few millimeters.

Gamma Rays. Gamma rays (γ) are highly penetrating electromagnetic radiations that travel at the speed of light (they are not particles and have no mass). They originate from transitions between energy levels in the nucleus.

Characteristic X Rays. Some radioactive decay processes result in the loss of an inner orbital electron from an atom. When outer electrons fill these inner vacancies, x rays whose energy is characteristic of that particular atom are emitted. These radiations differ from gamma rays only in their origin (electron orbits as opposed to nucleus) and are almost always of lower energy than gamma rays.

Types of Radioactive Decay

The particular mode of radioactive decay depends on the inherent "problem" of the unstable nucleus: whether there is only extra energy, or whether there are too many protons relative to the number of neutrons or vice versa. The decay proc-

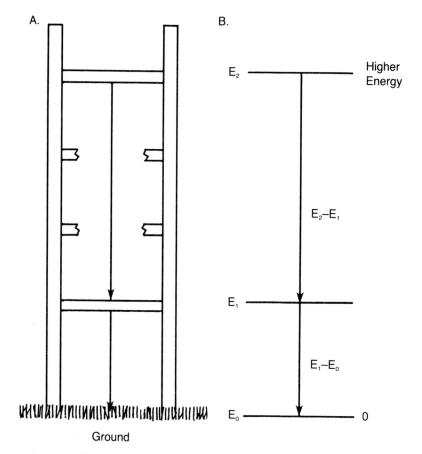

Fig. 2–1. *A.* A ladder is shown with only certain rungs present. Movement from a higher to a lower state would be between rungs. *B.* Similarly, transitions in energy from higher to lower levels occur as discrete energy differences between permitted energy levels (E_2–E_1, E_1–E_0, etc.). Energy changes are indicated by lines or arrows that are drawn straight down.

esses, as we shall see, result in the emission of particles or energy from the unstable atom as the atom seeks to achieve stability. Radionuclides may decay by any one process or a combination of five processes.

Alpha Decay. When the nucleus emits an alpha particle, the atomic number (Z) and atomic mass number (A) decrease by two and four, respectively. Radionuclides that decay by alpha emission are not important in nuclear medicine.

Beta Minus (β^-) Decay. Radioactive atoms that contain too many neutrons decay by the emission of negatively charged electrons called beta particles (β^-). These particles are emitted from the nu-

cleus and involve the conversion of a neutron (n) into a proton (p) and an electron (β^-).

$$n \rightarrow p + \beta^-$$

Though the mass number (A) of the nucleus remains unchanged, the number of protons increases by one so that a new element results. A gamma ray may or may not accompany beta emission. An example is the beta minus decay of radioactive P-32 ($T\frac{1}{2}$ = 14.3 days), which occurs directly from the excited state to the ground state (Fig. 2–3).

Gamma Decay (Isomerism). Gamma decay does not involve the emission of particles or a change in the number of protons

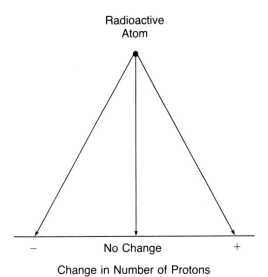

Fig. 2–2. Nuclear decay scheme; an arrow straight down indicates a change in energy only. An arrow slanting down to the left indicates a reduction in the number of protons, while an arrow slanting down to the right indicates an increase in the number of protons.

or neutrons. The nucleus changes only in its energy status, from higher to lower, by emitting a gamma ray photon. In most instances, the radioactive (or "excited") state of a nucleus is very short ($<10^{-10}$ sec), but occasionally this time is prolonged to minutes or hours. When this prolonged transition state occurs, the radionuclide is

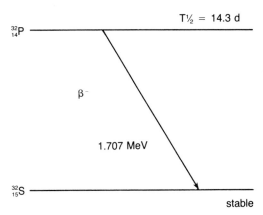

Fig. 2–3. The decay scheme of P-32. It should be noted that because of the change in atomic numbers, the product atom is *chemically different* from the parent atom. Other important radionuclides that decay by beta minus decay include Mo-99, Fe-59, Xe-133, and I-131.

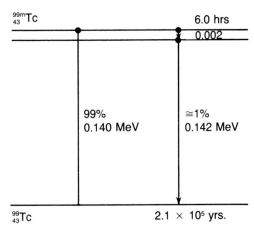

Fig. 2–4. The decay scheme of Tc-99m. The percentages indicate the fraction of the time each type of emission occurs. Approximately 10% of the 140 KeV gamma rays are internally converted to electrons.

called *metastable* (indicated by adding an "m" to the mass number), and the nuclide pair are called *isomers*. For example, Mo-99 decays by emission of a beta particle to Tc-99m, which is metastable and decays with a half-life of 6 hours, by gamma emission, to Tc-99 (Tc-99m and Tc-99 are isomers).

$$\text{Mo-99} \xrightarrow[\beta^-]{86\%} \text{Tc-99m} \xrightarrow{\text{I.T.}} \text{Tc-99}$$

Mo-99   Tc-99m   Tc-99
67 hr   6.0 hr 2.1×10^5 yr
└──────── 14% ────────┘

The decay scheme for the isomeric transition of Tc-99m to Tc-99 is shown in Figure 2–4. The percentages in Figure 2–4 indicate what portion of the decaying atoms follows each route (this is called "branching"). Obviously, almost all Tc-99m atoms emit the 140 KeV photon.*

Internal conversion is a process that competes with gamma ray emission. Under some circumstances, excess energy that would ordinarily be emitted as a gamma ray is transferred to an inner atomic electron, which is then emitted. Characteristic x rays are also emitted after internal con-

---

*One KeV is the amount of energy equal to the kinetic energy acquired by an electron accelerated through a potential difference of 1 volt. The KeV equals 1000 eV, while an MeV of energy equals 1000 KeV, or 1,000,000 eV.

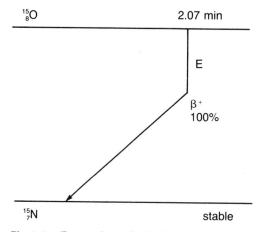

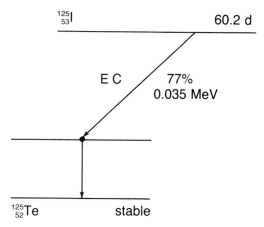

Fig. 2–5. Decay scheme for O-15, a positron emitter with a half-life of 2.07 minutes. The energy interval E represents the energy required to convert a proton to a neutron in the nucleus (1.02 MeV).

Fig. 2–6. Decay scheme for I-125. Since the 35.5 KeV gamma ray is 80% internally converted to electrons, most of the detectable radiations are characteristic x rays.

version as outer electrons "fall in" to fill the hole in the inner shell. Internal conversion is important to nuclear medicine because it (1) decreases the number of gamma rays for counting and imaging and (2) increases the radiation dose to the patient (emitted electrons contribute significantly to local tissue radiation exposure).

Positron Decay. Positron (β^+) decay occurs in nuclei that have an excess number of protons and have sufficient energy to convert a proton in the nucleus to a neutron. In this process, a positron is emitted.

$$p \rightarrow n + \beta^+$$

An example of the decay scheme with positron emission is O-15 (Fig. 2–5). When positrons are emitted from the nuclei of proton-rich radionuclides, they lose energy over a very small distance and then interact with a negative electron in a nearby atom. At the moment of this interaction (called "annihilation"), two gamma rays are emitted in opposite directions, each with an energy of 511 KeV. These gamma rays may be used for certain types of imaging with special types of radiation detection devices, called PETT (Positron Emission Transmission Tomography) units. Radionuclides used in medicine that decay by

positron emission include C-11, N-13, and F-18.

Electron Capture. An alternative method of decay for proton-rich radionuclides is electron capture (EC). In this process, the nucleus "captures" an inner orbital electron, converting a proton in the nucleus into a neutron.

$$p + e^- \rightarrow n$$

As outer electrons fall in to fill inner electron shell vacancies, characteristic x rays are emitted. I-125 is an example of a radionuclide that decays by electron capture (Fig. 2–6). Other radionuclides presently used in nuclear medicine that decay by electron capture include I-123, Yb-169, Ga-67, In-111, Cr-51, Co-57, Xe-127, and Tl-201.

Decay Data and Abundance. Decay information for gamma-emitting radionuclides important in clinical nuclear medicine has been compiled in Table 2–1.

2.6   UNITS OF RADIOACTIVITY

Amounts of radioactivity (activity) are expressed in units called *curies*. The initial definition of a curie was based upon the rate of decay of radium, which was thought (incorrectly) to be 3.7×10^{10} disintegra-

Table 2–1.   Decay data for gamma-emitting radionuclides important in nuclear medicine.

Radionuclide	Physical Half-life		Decay Mode	Primary Photon		
				Energies (KeV)		% Abundance*
C-11	20.3	min	β⁺	511		199
N-13	10	min	β⁺	511		200
O-15	2.0	min	β⁺	511		200
F-18	110	min	β⁺	511		194
Cr-51	27.8	days	EC	5	(x ray)	0.22
				324		10
Co-57	270	days	EC	14		10
				122		86
				136		10
Fe-59	45	days	β⁻	1100		56
				1290		44
Ga-67	78.1	hr	EC	93		38
				185		24
				300		16
Se-75	120	days	EC	121		16
				136		54
				265		57
				280		24
				400		12
Tc-99m	6	hr	IT	18	(x ray)	6.5
				140		88
In-111	2.81	days	EC	172		90
				247		94
I-123	13	hr	EC	27	(x ray)	71
				159		84
I-125	60.2	days	EC	27	(x ray)	115
				31	(x ray)	25
				35		7
I-131	8	days	β⁻	284		6
				364		82
				637		7
Xe-127	36.4	days	EC	172		25
				203		68
				375		17
Xe-133	5.3	days	β⁻	31	(x ray)	39
				81		36
Yb-169	31.8	days	EC	50	(x ray)	119
				63		45
				131		11
				177		17
				198		26
				308		11
Tl-201	73.1	hr	EC	69–80	(x rays)	10
				135		3
				167		95

*Relative number of emissions per disintegration expressed as a percentage. Thus, if the abundance is 100%, one photon of that particular energy would be emitted per atomic disintegration. (From MIRD Pamphlet 10. Dillman, LT, Von der Lage, FC. Radionuclide decay schemes and nuclear parameters for use in radiation-dose estimation. New York, Society of Nuclear Medicine, 1975, with permission.)

tions/second (dps) per gram (Ra-226). This definition has remained and is now applied to other radionuclides.

Because the curie is so large, the millicurie (1/1000 of a curie) and the microcurie (1/1,000,000 of a curie) are more frequently used in nuclear medicine and pharmacy.

$$1 \text{ curie (Ci)} = 3.7 \times 10^{10} \text{ dps}$$

$$1 \text{ millicurie (mCi)} = 3.7 \times 10^{7} \text{ dps}$$

$$1 \text{ microcurie } (\mu\text{Ci}) = 3.7 \times 10^{4} \text{ dps}$$

A new unit of activity, the Becquerel (Bq), has been proposed (1 Bq = 1 disintegration/sec). Because the Becquerel and other proposed units of the International System (SI units) are not widely used, this book retains the units currently employed (i.e., curie, millicurie, and microcurie).

2.7 RADIOACTIVE DECAY AND HALF-LIFE

Unlike the shelf lives of ordinary pharmaceuticals, which are limited by chemical degradation, the useful lifetimes of radiopharmaceuticals are usually determined by radioactive decay, which constantly decreases the amount of radioactivity present. Thus, when compounding or using radiopharmaceuticals, one must be able to calculate the amount of radioactivity present at any given time. This determination can be made in two ways: by plotting activity remaining against time elapsed, or by calculating using the "decay" formula.

Physical Half-Life

Since the decay (or decrease) in the number of atoms is an exponential process, the decay can be plotted on a log-linear graph to yield a straight line. Figure 2–7 shows the decay of three radionuclides (activity plotted against time). The value given with each radionuclide is the time required for activity to reach half of its original value, the *physical half-life*. Note in Figure 2–7 that

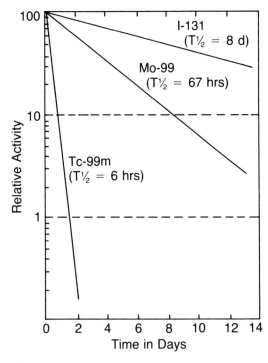

Fig. 2–7. Decay of Tc-99m, Mo-99, and I-131 plotted on a semilogarithmic graph. Half-lives are shown in parentheses.

as the physical half-life becomes shorter, the slope of the line becomes steeper, and the decay occurs more rapidly. Thus, knowing the elapsed time, the fraction remaining can be read directly from a decay plot.

Calculation. The fraction of a radionuclide remaining can also be determined by calculations using the "exponential decay law:"

$$\text{Fraction remaining} = e^{-\lambda t}$$

where λ is the decay constant (the fraction decaying per unit time), t is the time over which the decay occurs, and e is the base of the natural logarithm (2.7183). Values for e are shown in Appendix A. The decay constant λ can be computed using the following relationship to the half-life ($T\frac{1}{2}$):

$$T\tfrac{1}{2} = 0.693/\lambda$$

EXAMPLE
A syringe containing 10 mCi of Tc-99m ($T\frac{1}{2}$ = 6 hr) cannot be used until 4 hours later. At that

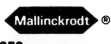

Diagnostic Products Division
Mallinckrodt, Inc.
St. Louis, MO 63134

352

IODINATED I 125 ALBUMIN INJECTION
IHSA I 125 ISOJEX™ Syringe

Act.	1 0 µCi/Syringe
As of 12 Noon CT	
Vol.	1 A P R 8 5
	1 . 5 ml
No. Syringes	1 0
Sp. Act.	8 . 5 µCi/mg
Exp. Date	2 8 M A Y 8 5
Lot	3 5 2 5 0 0 2

DIAGNOSTIC   Sterile, Pyrogen-Free Solution
For Intravenous Administration Store at 2°C. to 8°C.

Prepared from a licensed and released lot of Albumin Human.
Each ml contains:

Albumin Human	0.8 mg
Sodium Chloride	9 mg
Diabasic Sodium Phosphate Anhydrous	122 µg
Monobasic Potassium Phosphate	64 µg
Guanidine Hydrochloride	0.5 µg

Benzyl Alcohol 0.9%, v/v, added as a preservative. Sodium Hydroxide or Hydrochloric Acid may be present for pH adjustment.

(For information on dosage, administration and indications see package insert.)

CAUTION: Federal (U.S.A.) law prohibits dispensing without prescription.

WARNING Radioactive drugs must be handled only by qualified personnel in conformity with regulations of the U.S. Nuclear Regulatory Commission, state regulatory agencies where applicable, or other regulatory agencies authorized to license the use of radionuclides.

CAUTION

RADIOACTIVE MATERIAL

Attention-Produits Radioactif

R4/83   Canadian License No. 129

Fig. 2–8. Product labeling for ^{125}I-albumin injection. This radiopharmaceutical is prepared in unit dose syringes for intravenous administration. Note that the activity concentration and the specific activity are shown for this particular radiopharmaceutical.

time, how much Tc-99m remains? First, λ is calculated for Tc-99m

$$\lambda = 0.693/T\tfrac{1}{2} = 0.693/6 = 0.116/hr$$

Four hours later, the fraction remaining, $e^{-\lambda t}$, may be calculated as follows:

$$e^{-\lambda t} = e^{-(0.116)(4)} = e^{-0.464}$$

Using the e^{-x} table (see Appendix A) for e value of $x = 0.464$,

$$e^{-x} = 0.632$$

Thus, the initial 10 mCi of Tc-99m has decayed to

$$10 \text{ mCi} \times 0.632 = 6.32 \text{ mCi}$$

The activity required in order to have a specific amount of activity present at some future time can also be determined by calculation. In such a "precalibration" calculation, the activity desired at some future time is *divided* by the fraction of activity that would remain if decay had occurred over that same time interval.

EXAMPLE

Using the previous problem as a basis, we might desire to know how much Tc-99m should be placed within a syringe to have 10 mCi 4 hours *later*. As previously calculated, the fraction of Tc-99m activity remaining after 4 hours' decay is 0.632. Thus, the "precalibration" amount can be determined using the following simple calculation:

Activity/Fraction remaining

$$= 10 \text{ mCi}/0.632 = 15.8 \text{ mCi}$$

Thus, 15.8 mCi must be placed in the syringe to have 10 mCi remaining 4 hours later.

2.8 SPECIFIC ACTIVITY AND CONCENTRATION

Specific activity is defined as the amount of radioactivity per unit mass of a radionuclide or a labeled compound. Specific activity is usually expressed in units such as mCi/mg, Ci/g, or Ci/mole and is often provided on the manufacturer's product label (Fig. 2–8).

Activity concentration is defined as the amount of radioactivity per unit volume (mCi/ml). Since most radiopharmaceuticals are liquids (either solutions or suspensions), the amount of radioactivity per volume (activity concentration) must be known for a given time in order that the desired amount of radioactivity may be dispensed. For instance, if a 20-mCi dose is requested and the radiopharmaceutical activity concentration is presently 32 mCi/ml, approximately 0.62 ml must be dispensed to provide the necessary radioactivity.

Calculate:

$$\frac{\text{Activity Needed}}{\text{Activity Concentration*}} = \frac{20 \text{ mCi}}{32 \text{ mCi/ml}} = 0.62 \text{ ml}$$

REFERENCES

1. Chandra, R: Introductory Physics in Nuclear Medicine. Philadelphia, Lea & Febiger, 1976.
2. Dillman, LT, Von der Lage, FC: MIRD Pamphlet 10. Radionuclide Decay Schemes and Nuclear Parameters for Use in Radiation-Dose Estimation. New York, Society of Nuclear Medicine, 1975.
3. Sorenson, JA, Phelps, ME: Physics in Nuclear Medicine, New york, Grune and Stratton, 1980.

---

*Using the exponential decay law, fraction remaining = $e^{-\lambda t}$, the activity concentration can be calculated for any point in time as long as an initial activity concentration for a given time is known.

3

Production of Radioactivity

3.1 ORIGIN OF RADIONUCLIDES

Radionuclides that occur in nature are considered "natural" radioactivity. With few exceptions, such radionuclides are among the heaviest elements and are not useful in medicine. All radionuclides used today in medicine are artificially produced.

Man-made radionuclides are produced by bombarding the nuclei of stable atoms with subatomic particles (such as neutrons or protons) to make them unstable and radioactive. This process, which is called *nuclear reaction* or *activation*, can be produced by three methods:

1. proton bombardment
2. neutron bombardment
3. fission production

Proton Bombardment. Positively charged protons may be accelerated to energies sufficient for them to enter the nuclei of atoms in spite of the positive nuclear charge that repels them. Such a reaction (the entry of a proton into the nucleus) is likely to "knock out" a neutron, leaving the nucleus with excess energy (excited) and altered from its original structure. Since the proton replaces a neutron in the atom, the nucleus is considered *proton rich* (or neutron deficient). The cyclotron is the most common device used to accelerate protons.

Neutron Bombardment. Stable nuclei can be bombarded with low-energy neutrons in a nuclear reactor. When these nuclei "capture" a neutron, they possess excess energy by virtue of having too many neutrons and are said to be *neutron rich*.

Fission Products. When U-235 is bombarded with neutrons, excited (radioactive) nuclei are produced as a result of the fissioning, or splitting, of the now unstable U-235 atoms. The fission products formed possess more neutrons than are required for nuclear stability.

3.2 NUCLEAR NOMENCLATURE

The convention for expressing nuclear reactions in "shorthand" is:

$$\text{Target} \left(\begin{array}{cc} \text{Bombarding} & \text{Product} \\ \text{Particle,} & \text{Emission} \end{array} \right) \text{Product} \atop \text{Nucleus}$$

For example, the reaction whereby a stable atom X is bombarded with a neutron (n) to form a "compound nucleus" from which a proton (p) is immediately emitted to yield radioactive atom Y, can be written by the following nomenclature:

$$X (n, p) Y$$

3.3 NEUTRON/PROTON BALANCE

As stated in Chapter 2, the property of radioactivity results from imbalances that occur in the proton to neutron ratio. For nuclear stability, relatively more neutrons are required as atoms become larger and more complex. After particle bombardment, the number of protons or neutrons in the nucleus is changed and the new neutron to proton ratio determines the decay mode. Figure 3–1 shows a plot of the stable nuclides according to the number of pro-

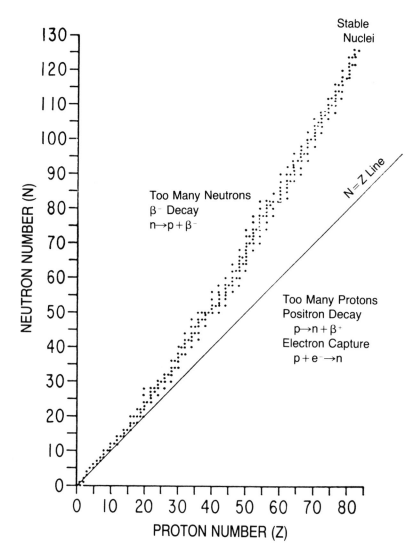

Fig. 3–1. Proton-neutron plot of stable nuclei (represented by dots). The 45-degree line indicates equal numbers of protons and neutrons (note the gradual increase in the numbers of neutrons relative to protons). Radionuclides above the stable elements will decay by negative beta decay while those below will decay by positron emission or electron capture. (From Quimby, EH, Feitelberg, S, Gross, W: Radioactive Nuclides in Medicine and Biology. Philadelphia, Lea & Febiger, 1970, p. 15.)

tons and neutrons present. Any radio-nuclide above the line of stability (such as neutron-rich products from nuclear reactors) would most likely decay by β⁻ decay. On the other hand, proton-rich radionuclides (which are produced in cyclotrons) lie below the line of stability and generally decay by electron capture or positron emission.

3.4 CARRIER

During target bombardment, not all of the stable atoms in the target are made radioactive. Therefore, the final product may contain, in addition to the product radionuclide, stable atoms (so-called carrier). The presence of carrier atoms in a product depends largely upon the radionuclide production process.

The term "carrier" arose from radiochemical processes in which small amounts of short-lived radionuclides could be precipitated ("carried down") by adding large amounts of a stable isotope in the same chemical form. There is, at present, confusion about whether any radionuclide can actually be carrier free, since minute amounts of stable atoms may occur in products by means other than product reactions. Suggestions for a less ambiguous nomenclature have been made by Wolf:

1. *Carrier-free* (CF) would apply to a radionuclide that is not contaminated with a stable or radioactive nuclide of the same element.
2. *No carrier added* (NCA) would apply to an element or compound to which no carrier of the same element has been intentionally or otherwise added during preparation.
3. *Carrier added* (CA) would apply to any element or compound to which a known amount of carrier has been added.

The "no carrier added" (NCA) designation would apply to most of the elements and compounds to which the term "carrier-free" is now applied.

3.5 ACCELERATOR-PRODUCED RADIONUCLIDES

Accelerators are devices that accelerate *subatomic charged* particles such as protons, deuterons (^{2}H nuclei), tritons (^{3}H nuclei), and alpha particles to very high energies (10 to 30 MeV). High energies are necessary since positively charged particles are repelled by the intense repulsive force associated with the positive charge of the protons in the atomic nuclei they are bombarding. Thus, positively charged particles must literally be "fired" into stable atoms to penetrate their nuclei. The two major types of particle accelerators are cyclotrons and linear accelerators.

Cyclotrons. These devices consist of a pair of hollow metal electrodes (called "dees" because they are shaped like the letter D) positioned between the poles of an electromagnet (Fig. 3–2). The dees are coupled to a high frequency electrical system so that the charge on each alternates more than a million times each second between positive and negative. The magnetic field is perpendicular (up and down) through the dees. A charged particle such as a proton or deuteron will be alternately repelled by the dee it is in and attracted to the other. The magnetic field acting perpendicular to the direction of motion of the charged particle bends the path to a circle. The result is a rapid acceleration of the particle as it spirals outward. The stream of high-energy particles produced can bombard an inner target or emerge from an outer window to bombard an outer target. Occasionally, neutrons may be desired for target bombardment in cyclotrons. This can be accomplished indirectly by bombarding a beryllium target with deuterons to produce neutrons.

Sorenson and Phelps have summarized the general characteristics of cyclotron-produced radionuclides:

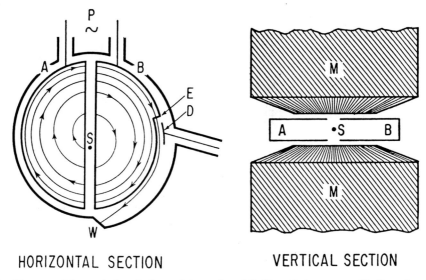

HORIZONTAL SECTION   VERTICAL SECTION

Fig. 3–2. Diagram of the central part of a cyclotron. A and B, Dees; S, ion source; P, alternating potential; D, deflecting plate; E, exit slit; W, window; MM, magnet plots. (From Quimby, EH, Feitelberg, S, Gross, W.: Radioactive Nuclides in Medicine and Biology. Philadelphia, Lea & Febiger, 1970, p. 37.)

1. Because a positive charge is added to the nucleus, cyclotron-produced radionuclides tend to decay by electron capture and positron production.
2. Addition of a positive charge to the target nucleus changes the atomic number and chemical properties of the target nucleus (i.e., nuclear transmutation), thus allowing complete separation of target and product atoms (carrier-free state). Product radionuclides, therefore, have very high specific activities.
3. Cyclotrons generally produce low "beam intensities" and, consequently, small quantities of radioactivity that are usually more expensive than radionuclides produced by other means (i.e., reactor-produced radionuclide).

Linear Accelerators. Linear accelerators, like cyclotrons, are devices that accelerate charged particles such as electrons, protons, and deuterons. Acceleration by increasing voltage occurs along a linear (rather than circular) path.

Radionuclides commonly used in medicine that are produced in cyclotrons are shown in Table 3–1.

3.6 REACTOR-PRODUCED RADIONUCLIDES

Another major source of artificial radionuclides is the nuclear reactor. Reactors serve as sources of neutrons and are dependent upon a process called nuclear fission for the production of neutrons. Within reactors, radioactive atoms are produced by two types of processes—fission and neutron bombardment.

Fission. The most widely used fissionable material is a naturally occurring isotope of uranium, U-235. When a U-235 nucleus captures a neutron, the resulting nucleus is very unstable and promptly breaks ("fissions") into two smaller atoms (fission fragments), more neutrons, and energy. In the reaction, the neutrons released are capable of bombarding other U-235 nuclei to produce additional fissions, which can lead to a self-sustaining nuclear chain reaction. When the reaction process is controlled and sustained at a desired level, as occurs at a nuclear power plant,

Table 3–1.   Some cyclotron-produced radionuclides used in nuclear medicine. (From Sorenson, JA, Phelps, ME: Physics in Nuclear Medicine. New York, Grune and Stratton, 1980. By permission.)

Product	Decay Mode	Common Production Reaction
C-11	β^+	$^{10}B(d,n)^{11}C$
		$^{11}B(p,n)^{11}C$
N-13	β^+	$^{12}C(d,n)^{13}N$
O-15	β^+	$^{14}N(d,n)^{15}O$
F-18	β^+, EC	$^{20}Ne(d,\alpha)^{18}F$
Na-22	β^-, EC	$^{23}Na(p,2n)^{22}Na$
K-43	β^-,γ	$^{40}Ar(\alpha,p)^{43}K$
Ga-67	EC,γ	$^{68}Zn(p,2n)^{67}Ga$
In-111	EC,γ	$^{109}Ag(\alpha,2n)^{111}In$
		$^{111}Cd(p,n)^{111}In$
I-123	EC,γ	$^{122}Te(d,n)^{123}I$
		$^{127}I(p,5n)^{123}Xe \xrightarrow{EC} {}^{123}I$
Xe-127	EC,γ	$^{133}Cs(p,2p5n)^{127}Xe$
Tl-201	EC,γ	$^{201}Hg(d,2n)^{201}Tl$
		$^{203}Tl(p,3n)^{201}Pb \xrightarrow{EC} {}^{201}Tl$

d—deuteron
n—neutron
α—alpha particle
p—proton

the energy emitted through fission may be used to generate power. Several of the fission fragments, the highly radioactive waste products of this process, are also useful in medicine.

The element uranium exists in nature chiefly as two isotopes, U-238 (99.3%) and U-235 (0.7%). Because U-238 is not fissionable, the fuel rods in reactor cores are typically made up of uranium that has an enriched U-235 content. Since U-235 is particularly fissionable by slow neutrons, fuel rods are surrounded by a "moderator" (usually water, heavy water, or graphite) whose purpose is to slow the neutrons to thermal energies. The result of fission occurring in the fuel rods is a large number of neutrons (called a high "flux") at the center of the reactor. Pneumatic sample lines lead to the reactor core for insertion of samples for neutron bombardment (Fig. 3–3).

Radionuclides may be obtained from the radioactive fission fragments when uranium fuel elements are periodically replaced (Fig. 3–4). Chemical separation techniques (precipitation techniques, solvent extraction, chromatography, etc.) are used to isolate certain radionuclides. Since in the fission process radionuclides of entirely new elements are formed (no stable elements or uranium remain after chemical separation), the fission product nuclei are usually carrier free with specific activities that are quite high. Fission product nuclei are usually neutron rich and decay by β^- emission.

Neutron Bombardment. Because the neutron has no electrical charge, there is no resistance to its entrance into the positively charged nucleus. When bombarding neutrons are captured by stable target nuclei, the most common result is an (n,γ) reaction that results in the production of neutron-rich radionuclides. The quantity of radioactive material produced depends upon the intensity of the neutron flux (i.e., the number of neutrons being "beamed" into the stable target), neutron energy, and the probability of neutron absorption by the target atoms. This probability of absorption (i.e., neutron activation) is called the "cross section" and is measured in units called "barns" (10^{-24} cm^2). The higher this value, the more readily neutron activation occurs. Sorenson and Phelps have

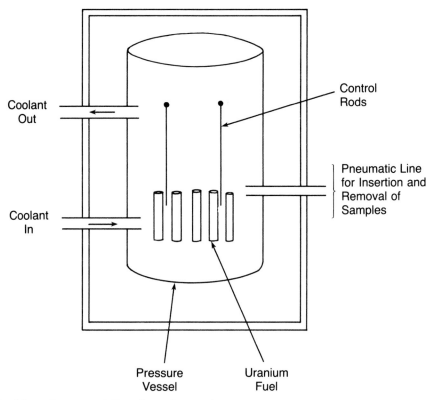

Fig. 3–3. Schematic representation of a nuclear reactor.

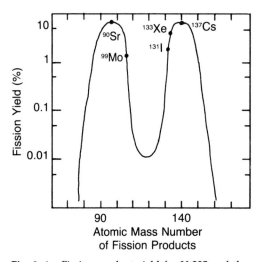

Fig. 3–4. Fission product yield for U-235 and thermal neutrons.

summarized the general characteristics of radionuclides produced by neutron bombardment:

1. Because neutrons are added to the nucleus, the products are generally neutron rich, lie above the line of stability (Fig. 3–1), and decay by β^- emission.

2. Since the (n,γ) reaction is the most common, the products of this reaction are not carrier free (they are radioisotopes of the target material and have the same atomic number). For this reason, radionuclides produced by neutron activation have very low specific activities.

3. Even with intense neutron fluxes, only a small portion of the target nuclei are activated (perhaps 1 in a million or less). Thus, (n,γ) products are of low specific activity.

Commonly used radionuclides that are

Table 3–2.   Some reactor-produced radionuclides used in nuclear medicine. (From Sorenson, JA, Phelps, ME: Physics in Nuclear Medicine. New York, Grune and Stratton, 1980. By permission.)

Radionuclide	Decay Mode	Production Reaction	σ (b)*
C-14	β^-	$^{14}N(n,p)^{14}C$	1.81
Na-24	β^-,γ	$^{23}Na(n,\gamma)^{24}Na$	0.53
P-32	β^-	$^{31}P(n,\gamma)^{32}P$	0.19
		$^{32}S(n,p)^{32}P$	—
S-35	β^-	$^{35}Cl(n,p)^{35}S$	—
K-42	β^-,γ	$^{41}K(n,\gamma)^{42}K$	1.2
Cr-51	EC,γ	$^{50}Cr(n,\gamma)^{51}Cr$	17
Fe-59	β^-,γ	$^{58}Fe(n,\gamma)^{59}Fe$	1.1
Se-75	EC,γ	$^{74}Se(n,\gamma)^{75}Se$	30
I-125	EC,γ	$^{124}Xe(n,\gamma)^{125}Xe\xrightarrow{EC}{}^{125}I$	110
I-131	β^-,γ	$^{130}Te(n,\gamma)^{131}Te\xrightarrow{\beta^-}{}^{131}I$	0.24

*Thermal neutron capture cross section, expressed in barns (σ) for (n,γ) reactions.
n—neutron
p—proton

prepared by neutron bombardment are given in Table 3–2.

3.7   YIELD OF RADIONUCLIDES

Occasionally, it is useful to calculate the yield of a particle bombardment reaction. The amount of radioactivity produced depends on the intensity (and energy) of the incident particles, the amount of target material, the half-life of the product nuclide, and the duration of the bombardment.

The activity (A) of a radionuclide being produced by particle bombardment can be calculated from:

$$A = \frac{\phi N \sigma}{3.7 \times 10^{10}}(1 - e^{-\lambda t})$$

where

A = activity in curies
ϕ = neutron flux (n/cm²/sec)
N = number of target atoms
σ = absorption cross section in barns (10^{-24} cm²/atom)
λ = decay constant of product radionuclide
t = duration of radiation (sec)

The term $(1 - e^{-\lambda t})$ in the previous equation approaches unity when t is greater than about 4 half-lives, giving a saturation activity (A_s):

$$A_s = \frac{\phi N \sigma}{3.7 \times 10^{10}}$$

where A_s is the maximum activity in curies. When the bombardment time equals 1 half-life, half of the saturation activity (A_s) will be achieved (¾ this activity after 2 half-lives, and so on). Thus bombardment times beyond 3 to 4 half-lives are unproductive.

3.8   THE TARGET

Various types of targets have been designed and used in both reactors and cyclotrons. Certain requirements must be met in the practical use of target substances.

1. The target material for irradiation must be pure and preferably mono-isotopic, since extraneous nuclear reactions might otherwise occur, resulting in the production of an undesirable radioactive element.

2. Irradiation can cause temperature in the target as high as 1000°C. For this reason, the target is likely to burn unless a method of heat dissipation is established. Generally, some type of target cooling is employed, and most targets are designed as foil to maximize heat dissipation.

3.9   TARGET PROCESSING

Following irradiation, the target is usually dissolved in an appropriate solvent, and various chemical methods (solvent extraction, gel chromatography, ion exchange, distillation, and precipitation) are used to separate and purify the desired radioactive component.

3.10 RADIONUCLIDE GENERATORS

The imaging techniques currently used in nuclear medicine require high intensities of gamma ray photons in order to obtain high-resolution dynamic or static images. This need must be balanced with that of maintaining radiation doses acceptable to the patient. While the use of short-lived radionuclides satisfies both these requirements, supplying rapidly decaying radionuclides to users distant from the site of production may be a logistic problem. Specifically, the costs of production and delivery, as well as the uncertainty of air transportation, become important considerations in these situations. Radionuclide generators essentially eliminate the difficulties associated with the use of short-lived radionuclides.

A typical radionuclide generator consists of a longer-lived *parent* that decays to form a shorter-lived *daughter*. The radionuclide pair is contained in an apparatus that allows separation and removal of the daughter and retention of the parent. Within the generator, the short-lived daughter radionuclide is continually formed by decay of the parent.

A generator system should have the following properties:
1. It should be easy to operate.
2. The daughter must have high purity (chemical and radionuclide) and must be a different chemical element than the parent (i.e., not a radioisotope).
3. It must be sterile and pyrogen free.
4. The daughter product should be in a form convenient for radiopharmaceutical preparation.

Commercially prepared generators are sterilized, shielded, and automatic in operation (Fig. 3–5). The generator consists of a glass or plastic column containing an ion-exchange resin or alumina held in place by a fritted glass disk. The parent radionuclide is absorbed onto the ion-exchange column.

Since chemical properties of the daughter atoms are different from the parent atoms (β^-, β^+, and EC decay result in a change in proton number), separation is enhanced. Removal of the less tightly bound daughter from the column ("elution") is accomplished by the flow of the eluant (usually saline) through the column. A bacteriostatic agent may be added to the eluant or, more commonly, a millipore filter is attched to the end of the column in order to ensure sterility.

Radionuclide generators operate on the principle that the decay of a relatively long-lived parent continually produces a shorter-lived daughter. As the longer-lived parent decays, the activity associated with the daughter continues to increase until they are approximately equal, or at equilibrium. From this point, the daughter activity decreases at the rate that the parent decays. To understand the relationship of parent and daughter activity with time, we must consider the two types of equilibrium: secular and transient.

Secular equilibrium occurs when the parent's half-life is much longer than the daughter's; equilibrium effectively occurs after about 5 to 6 daughter half-lives. An example of secular equilibrium is shown in Figure 3–6. The following equation describes the relationship between initial parent (A_p) and daughter (A_d) activity at some later time, (t).

$$A_d = A_p \left(1 - e^{-\lambda t}\right)$$

Examples of radionuclide generators which operate on the basis of secular equilibrium include Sn-113/In-113m, Rb-81/Kr-81m, and Sr-82/Rb-82.

Transient equilibrium exists when the half-life of the parent is greater than the daughter by only a factor of 10 or less. Since the parent decays significantly during the half-

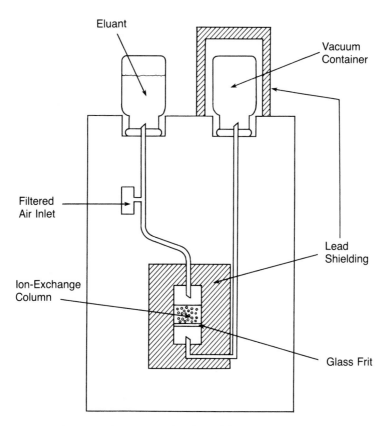

Fig. 3–5. Cross section of a "typical" commercial radionuclide generator.

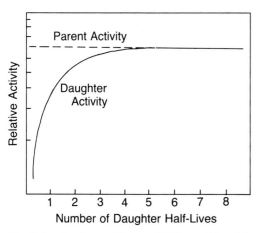

Fig. 3–6. Secular equilibrium. Build-up of daughter activity when $T_d \ll T_p$. Eventually, equilibrium is achieved, and the short-lived daughter appears to decay with the same half-life as the parent.

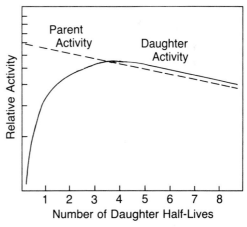

Fig. 3–7. Transient equilibrium occurs when $T_p > T_d$. This example shows build-up and decay of activity for $T_p = 10T_d$. Eventually, transient equilibrium is achieved when parent and daughter decay curves are parallel. (Daughter activity exceeds that of the parent only where all parent atoms (100%) decay to the daughter.)

life of the daughter, the parent's activity decreases significantly as the daughter's activity increases (Fig. 3–7), so that the daughter's activity at equilibrium may actually exceed that of the parent. At equilibrium, the amount of the daughter's activity is equal to that which decays, then decreases with an "apparent half-life" equal to the physical half-life of the parent. Transient equilibrium is reached when the ratio of the parent's to the daughter's activity remains constant. The ratio of parent to daughter at transient equilibrium is given by the following formula.

$$A_p/A_d = \frac{\lambda_d - \lambda_p}{\lambda_d}$$

The number of daughter atoms (N_d) present at any time (t) can also be calculated by

$$N_d = \frac{\lambda_p}{T_d - T_p} N_p (e^{-\lambda_p t} - e^{-\lambda_d t})$$

where N_p is the number of parent atoms present at t = 0. Since activity (A) is given by the relationship $A = N\lambda$, many atoms can be converted to activity. The most widely used generator is the Mo-99/Tc-99m generator, which operates on the principle of transient equilibrium.

REFERENCES

1. Chandra, R: Introductory Physics of Nuclear Medicine. Philadelphia, Lea & Febiger, 1976.
2. Dillman, LT, Von der Lage, FC: Radionuclide Decay Schemes and Nuclear Parameters for Use in Radiation-Dose Estimation. MIRD Pamphlet No. 10. New York, Society of Nuclear Medicine, 1975.
3. Quimby, EH, Feitelberg, S, Gross, W: Radioactive Nuclides in Medicine and Biology. Philadelphia, Lea & Febiger, 1970.
4. Sorenson, JA, Phelps, ME: Physics in Nuclear Medicine. New York, Grune and Stratton, 1980.
5. Wolf, AP: Letter to the Editor. J Nucl Med 22:392–393, 1981.

Instrumentation for the Detection and Measurement of Radioactivity

In nuclear medicine, several different types of radiation detection systems are used to ascertain the presence, type, and amount of radioactivity, as well as the quantity of radiation emitted. The operation of radiation detectors involves *ionization*, the process by which ionizing radiations dissipate their energy in matter (the process involves ejection of orbital electrons from stable atoms). The electrical charge of ionized atoms can be used to generate either electrical pulses (counts) or electrical current, allowing the detection and measurement of radioactivity. The types of detection systems are discussed in this chapter.

4.1 GAS-FILLED DETECTORS

The operation of gas-filled detectors is based upon the production of ionization-induced electrical currents within the gas cavities of such devices. Because the gas under ordinary circumstances acts as an insulator and constitutes a "break" in the circuit, there is no flow of current, even with voltage applied across the gas. Ionization of the gas by radiations, however, results in the production of ions and a measurable current flow (Fig. 4–1). The most common design for these detectors is a central wire (electrode) inside a cylinder. Ionization chambers and Geiger-Mueller (GM) counters are the most important gas-filled detectors and are used in nuclear medicine primarily as survey instruments

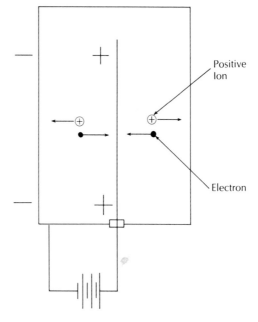

Fig. 4–1. Simple circuit for a gas-filled detector. Positive atoms and negative electrons liberated by ionizing radiation are collected by the positive and negative electrodes to produce a current flow in the circuit because of the voltage.

or as area monitors for the detection of small amounts of radioactivity.

4.2 IONIZATION CHAMBERS

Air or inert gases (such as argon under pressure) are used in ionization chamber detectors. In these devices, the voltage between electrodes is sufficient to collect all of the positive and negative ions produced. Since few ionizations are produced by a single ionizing ray or particle, however, it

29

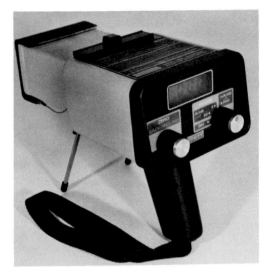

Fig. 4–2. An ionization chamber survey instrument. (Courtesy Keithley Instruments.)

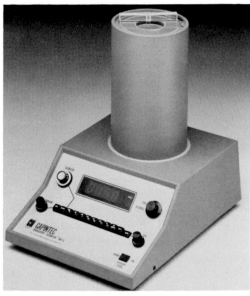

Fig. 4–3. A radionuclide dose calibrator. (Courtesy Capintec, Inc.)

is not usually possible to record these *individual* radiation events (i.e., "counts"). Instead, the total current produced by a large number of counts is measured either as the rate of charge production or as an accumulation of charge over time. Sensitive current measuring devices, called electrometers, convert these very small currents into measurements of either radiation exposure rates or amounts of radioactivity. The two major devices in nuclear medicine that use an ionization chamber-electrometer combination are the *survey meter* and the *radionuclide dose calibrator.*

Survey Meter. The ionization chamber survey instrument, commonly known as the "cutie-pie," consists of a large cylindrical outer portion with a central wire electrode (Fig. 4–2). Since ionization chambers collect all of the ions produced in the chamber, these devices are calibrated to read radiation exposure levels, usually in roentgen*/hour, which are displayed on a meter. These instruments are used to measure or monitor radiation levels from about 1 mR/

hr up to several R/hr and to determine exposure levels around large sources of radiation (e.g., shipments of radiopharmaceuticals, such as therapeutic amounts of radioiodine). Periodic calibration of survey instruments is essential to assure that the exposure level readings are accurate.

Radionuclide Dose Calibrators. These instruments (Fig. 4–3), which are employed to assay the *amounts* of radioactivity administered to patients, use an ionization chamber with a central "well" cavity large enough to accept syringes and vials (Fig. 4–3). The current produced in the chamber depends on the type and amount of radiation emitted. Because each radionuclide has characteristic decay patterns and photon emissions, equal activities of different radionuclides generate different current flows. For example, 1 mCi of Tc-99m does *not* produce the same amount of ionization current as 1 mCi of I-131. In order to permit the accurate assay of different radionuclides, most calibrators contain a voltage gain amplifier mechanism (Fig. 4–4), which produces different voltages to drive the output display for each radionuclide.

---

*The roentgen (R) is the unit of radiation exposure that refers to the amount of ionization produced in air by x rays or gamma rays. The milliroentgen (mR) is a smaller unit (1 mR = 1/1000 R).

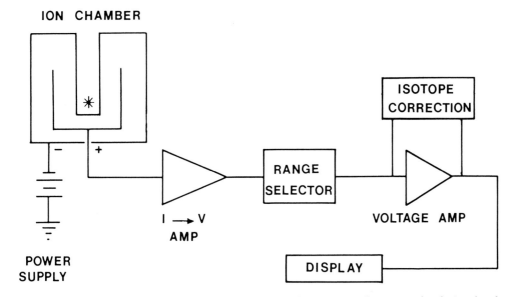

Fig. 4–4. Schematic of a radionuclide dose calibrator showing the power supply connected to the ion chamber, a current-to-voltage amplifier, a voltage gain amplifier, an isotope correction device to control the gain on the voltage gain amplifier, and an output display. Sample to be assayed (*). (From Kowalsky, RJ, Johnston, RE, and Chan, FH.: Dose calibrator performance and quality control. J Nucl Med Technol 5:36, 1977, with permission.)

The range selector switch selects different activity ranges, while the radionuclide correction box adjusts the gain of the voltage amplifier so that equal activities will produce the same reading.

Radionuclide dose calibrator accuracy may be affected by the type of radiopharmaceutical container (this is particularly true for radionuclides with low energy gamma emissions) as well as by changes in sample volumes. Effects of dilution of radioactivity (by changes in sample volume) should be determined so that appropriate correction factors can be applied if necessary. It is also important to verify the linearity of these devices, that is, the ability of a dose calibrator to accurately measure a wide range of activities (the test for linearity is done by periodic assay of a radionuclide such as Tc-99m as it decays over several half-lives). Tests for effects of sample volume upon radionuclide dose calibrator accuracy and dose calibrator linearity are discussed in Chapter 9.

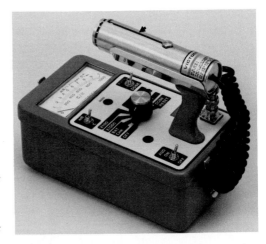

Fig. 4–5. A GM survey meter. The detecting tube *(arrow)* is usually covered with a sliding metal shield. Penetrating (gamma rays) and nonpenetrating (beta particles) radiations can be distinguished by observing the difference in count rates with and without the shield. (Courtesy Victoreen Instruments.)

4.3 GEIGER-MUELLER (GM) SURVEY METERS

These rugged instruments are useful in radiation protection (Fig. 4–5), primarily for area monitoring for radioactive contamination.

GM survey meters are highly sensitive and can be used to determine the presence of small amounts of radioactivity. They are hand held and most are equipped with earphones or audible beepers that further increase their detection sensitivity.

4.4   SCINTILLATION DETECTORS AND SPECTROMETERS

Solid scintillation crystal detectors were developed because gas-filled detectors are inefficient for detection of gamma rays and cannot distinguish radiation events of different energies.

Principles of Scintillation Detection. The most suitable scintillation detectors use a class of solids called "fluors," which have the property of fluorescence (giving off light) when they absorb radiation energy. These instruments get their name from the flash of light which is called a scintillation. Most of these fluor materials contain small quantities of impurity atoms or "activators" that are purposely added to produce usable scintillations. The most commonly used scintillator for detectors in nuclear medicine is sodium iodide activated with thallium, NaI(Tl).

When gamma rays interact in the NaI(Tl) crystal they lose energy and emit light (Fig. 4–6). The amount of energy lost in the crystal depends on the energy of the gamma ray photon and relates directly to the output of light from the crystal. This relationship allows energy-selective counting.

Light produced by the crystal is converted into electrical pulses by a device called a photomultiplier tube (PMT). In the PMT, pulses are multiplied to form a voltage output pulse that is directly proportional to gamma ray energy. Pulses are linearly increased in size by an amplifier and then sorted, according to size (and gamma ray energy), by a spectrometer.

The essential components of a spectrometer are two adjustable "discriminators," which can be used to select a "window" that determines the range of gamma ray energies (pulse sizes) that will be counted.

Scintillation detector/spectrometer systems can be used to measure *pulse-height* (gamma ray energy) *spectra*. These can be derived manually with a single channel analyzer by progressively advancing a narrow window up the energy scale and recording and plotting each count rate in turn. Multichannel analyzers (Fig. 4–7) use a digital storage device that receives and adds each pulse according to various energy channels (usually 512 or 1024 channels). Once the pulses are accumulated,

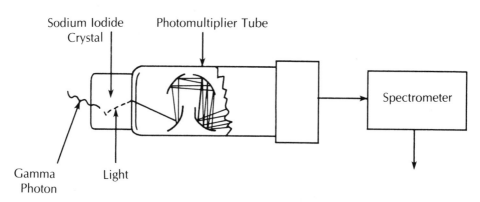

Fig. 4–6.   A diagram of a scintillation detector system. When gamma ray photons are absorbed in the scintillator, their energy is converted to light. In the photomultiplier tube, light is converted to electrons that are multiplied in number to form a voltage output pulse proportional to the light. The signal is then amplified, prior to pulse size analysis, by the spectrometer. Pulse size can be increased by increasing the high voltage on the photomultiplier tube or the amplifier gain.

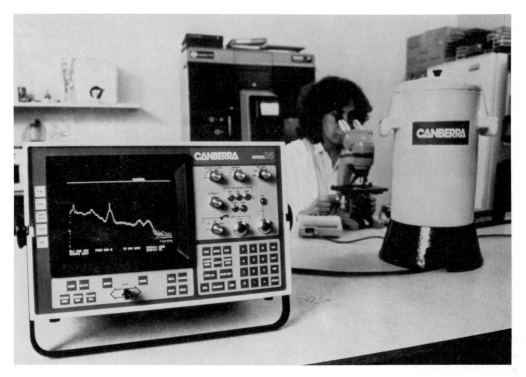

Fig. 4–7.   Multichannel analyzer with pulse-height spectrum shown on display. (Courtesy Canberra Instruments.)

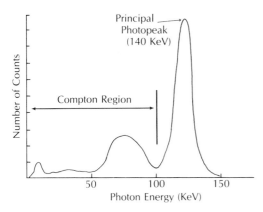

Fig. 4–8.   A pulse-height spectrum for Tc-99m. The principal photopeak occurs at 140 KeV.

multichannel analyzers display the spectrum on a cathode ray tube or other device.

When photons of a single energy strike a detector, the resulting pulse-height spectrum usually shows a total-absorption peak (the "photopeak"), resulting when photons impart all of their energy to the crystal, and a lower energy continuum (the "Compton-region"), produced when photons deposit only a part of their energy in the crystal (Fig. 4–8).

Scintillation Well Counter. The scintillation well/spectrometer is a vital part of the operation of the nuclear pharmacy; it is used for counting small samples of radioactivity. The well counter consists of an ordinary NaI(Tl) crystal with a hole at one end of the crystal for the insertion of the sample (Fig. 4–9). Lead shielding surrounding the detector reduces background radiation in well counters.

Gamma ray sources at a distance from a detector have a low counting efficiency since only a small fraction of emitted radiations reach the detector crystal. If the source is placed against the surface of the detector, half the emitted gamma rays strike the detector, but half are lost and cannot be counted (this is said to be "2π geometry"). When a source is placed inside

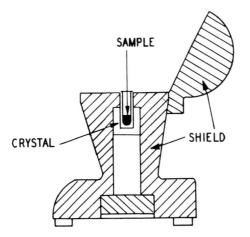

WELL TYPE SCINTILLATION DETECTOR

Fig. 4–9. The well-type scintillation detector with access hole to allow insertion of sample.

the detector, it is said to be counted in "4π geometry" (Fig. 4–10). Although some gamma rays are lost through the hole in the top of the well, the fraction lost depends upon the source position (it varies between 5% for sources at the bottom of the well and 50% for those at the top of the well). Thus, changes in sample volume can alter source position and can affect count rate significantly. For this reason, when comparing the activity of the two samples, the best approach is to use identical sample volumes. If this is not possible, a volume

correction factor can be obtained either by adding radioactive solution at a constant concentration or by diluting an initial radioactive sample with increasing volumes of water.

When two gamma rays emitted by the same radionuclide reach the detector simultaneously, they are recorded as a single event, and an extra peak appears on the energy spectrum, a so-called sum-coincidence peak. When samples are at some distance from the detector, such events are highly unlikely, but when a source is counted in a well system (particularly if the radioactivity levels are high), the probability that two coincident gamma rays will be counted is much higher ($\cong 100\%$). Thus, sum peaks are observed primarily with well counting. For example, when I-125 is counted in a well system, a 35.4 KeV gamma ray that strikes the detector crystal simultaneously with a 27 KeV x ray results in a 62.4 KeV sum peak (i.e., 35.4 KeV + 27 KeV = 62.4 KeV).

Counters require a period of time to record and process a pulse; this is called the *resolving time*. Although scintillation counters are considered to be "fast" among counters, counting excessively large amounts of radioactivity may result in "count-loss."

Solid-State Detectors. The semiconduc-

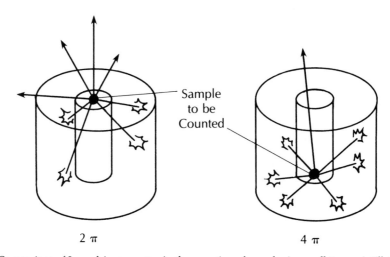

Fig. 4–10. Comparison of 2π and 4π geometry in the counting of samples in a well-type scintillation detector.

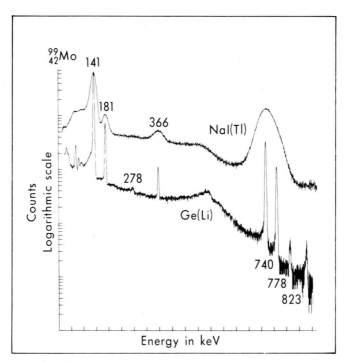

Fig. 4–11. Spectra of ^{99}Mo/^{99m}Tc gamma radiation as obtained with an NaI(Tl) spectrometer (upper spectrum) and a Ge(Li) spectrometer (lower spectrum). (From Raeside, DE, Widman, JC: An introduction to pulse electronics for nuclear medicine personnel. App. Rad. Jan–Feb 1977, pp. 199–205.)

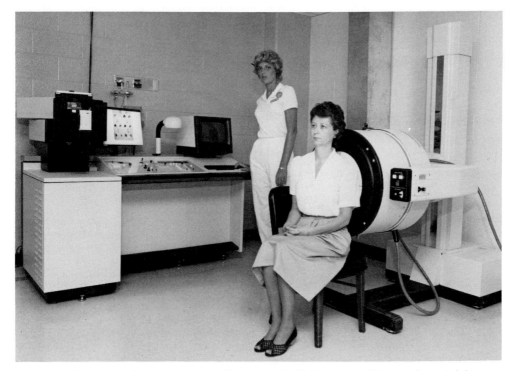

Fig. 4–12. Patient undergoing lung imaging with gamma scintillation camera. Patient is shown in left posterior oblique (LPO) position.

tor detector has been called a "solid-state ionization chamber." Although semiconductors are normally poor electrical conductors, the electrical charge that results from their ionization can be collected. The electrical signals produced by ionizing radiations are large, with small statistical fluctuations that improve energy resolution and make the photopeaks "sharper" than with NaI(Tl) crystals (Fig. 4–11). This allows the separation of radionuclides whose energies are close together. The most commonly used solid-state detector is the Ge(Li), or "lithium drifted germanium detector," in which the Li is added as an impurity to increase the signal output. Its major disadvantage is that Ge(Li) detectors must be stored and operated at liquid nitrogen temperature ($-196°C$). These systems are used in the nuclear pharmacy for high resolution identification of radionuclides by their gamma ray emissions.

4.5 CLINICAL SCINTILLATION IMAGING SYSTEMS

In nuclear medicine, images of radioactivity in body organs and vascular spaces are obtained using electronic systems that depict relative concentration by differences in film density.

Cameras. The gamma scintillation camera (Fig. 4–12) is a stationary device with a large NaI(Tl) crystal (usually ½ inch thick and up to 20 inches in diameter) that views *all* parts of a field rather than scanning the subject point-by-point. (The pictures from cameras should be called images or scintiphotos rather than scans.) The major advantage of cameras over scanners is their speed of image production, which also allows visualization of dynamic processes (such as organ blood flow) through the generation of multiple images over a very brief time.

Interactions of the gamma rays produce scintillations in the crystal; an array of at least 19 photomultiplier tubes views the scintillations and determines the position of the light impulse in the crystal (a pulse-height analyzer uses the sum of the intensities from all the tubes to determine energy). A cathode ray tube (CRT) briefly flashes at that point. Time exposures are recorded on film (Fig. 4–13). Because most scintillation camera crystals are relatively thin (½ inch or less), these detectors are not efficient for very high energy gamma rays ($\geq$ 300 KeV). With most crystals currently used, near-complete energy absorption occurs with gamma ray energies around 150 KeV.

Objects containing radioactivity are projected onto the crystal by radiations passing through the many holes in a lead collimator. The purpose of the collimator is to limit the field of view and to prevent radiations from nontarget areas from reaching the detector. Only those photons that originate below a hole in the collimator can interact with the crystal above that hole. Collimators can be of different sizes and shapes and may be classified as pinhole, high or low energy parallel hole, diverging, or converging (Fig. 4–14), depending on the thickness, shape, and size of the holes and on the way the objects are focused.

Scanners. The rectilinear scintillation scanner consists of a lead-shielded NaI(Tl) detector with a collimator in front of the crystal to focus the field of view to a small area directly beneath the crystal center. The detector is mounted on a rigid, motor-driven beam that drives the detector back and forth as the scanner maps out the distribution of activity within a body part (Fig. 4–15). The successive accumulation of information ("dots") can be seen as scan lines in the image. Images or "scans" from these devices may be life-sized or minified. For the most part, these devices have been replaced by gamma scintillation cameras.

Resolution and Sensitivity. Two concepts important to imaging should be mentioned at this point: *sensitivity*, which relates count rate and imaging time, and

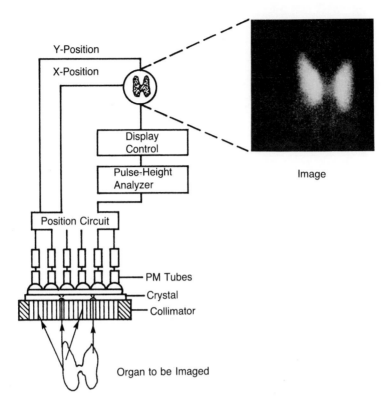

Fig. 4–13. Schematic of the basic components of image formation of the scintillation camera.

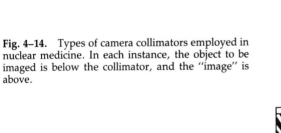

Fig. 4–14. Types of camera collimators employed in nuclear medicine. In each instance, the object to be imaged is below the collimator, and the "image" is above.

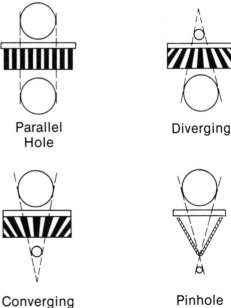

Parallel Hole

Diverging

Converging

Pinhole

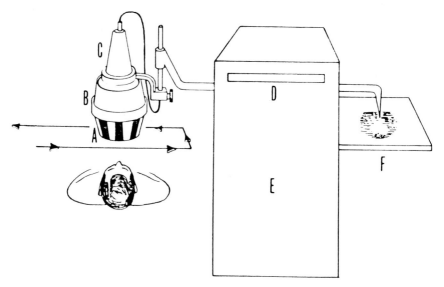

Fig. 4–15. Schematic of a mechanical rectilinear scanner. (A) Collimator. (B) Scintillation detecting unit. (C) Photomultiplier tube. (D) Photorecorder. (E) Processing unit. (F) "Dot" recording unit. (From Maynard, CD: Clinical Nuclear Medicine. Philadelphia, Lea & Febiger, 1969.)

resolution, which is the ability of the system to faithfully reproduce the radioactive object in the scintillation image. In general, resolution and sensitivity are determined to a great extent by the choice of lead collimator. For any same imaging interval, one achieves a higher sensitivity (count rate) at the cost of a reduction in image quality (loss of resolution), and vice versa. Thus, a high-resolution collimator with small holes will produce lower count rates, while a collimator designed to produce high sensitivity ("high efficiency collimators") must give up resolution in order to achieve high count rates.

Image Recording. Two film types are used to record images in clinical nuclear medicine—*transparent* film and *Polaroid* film. When transparent film is used, areas of radioactivity appear dark, while with Polaroid images the reverse is true. The thyroid image in Figure 4–13 was recorded on Polaroid film.

REFERENCES

1. Chandra, R: Introductory Physics of Nuclear Medicine. Philadelphia, Lea & Febiger, 1976.
2. Kowalsky, RJ, Johnston, RE, Chan, FH: Dose calibrator performance and quality control. J Nucl Med Technol 5:35–40, 1977.
3. Rollo, FD: Nuclear Medicine Physics, Instrumentation, and Agents. St. Louis, C.V. Mosby Company, 1977.
4. Sorenson, JA, Phelps, ME: Physics in Nuclear Medicine, New York, Grune and Stratton, 1980.

CHAPTER

5

Basics of Clinical Selection of Radiopharmaceuticals

When evaluating radiopharmaceuticals for clinical use, many factors must be taken into account. Among the preliminary characteristics, to be reviewed in the selection process are nuclear properties and biological behavior.

5.1 DESIRABLE NUCLEAR PROPERTIES

Principal Photon Energy. Principal photon energy is a critical factor in the clinical application of radiopharmaceuticals because it largely determines detection characteristics (Fig. 5–1). Ideally, a gamma photon energy of approximately 150 KeV is desirable, since this energy results in nearly complete deposition within the standard scintillation crystal of most camera systems. While photon energies greater than 150 KeV can be imaged, the detection sensitivity of the gamma scintillation camera *decreases* substantially with much higher photon energies. Higher photon energies also require the use of thicker-walled collimators, decreasing the number of photons that can be detected. Very low energy photons, on the other hand, may be attenuated by body tissues and hence not be detectable externally.

The radionuclide used for imaging should also be monoenergetic; that is, gamma photons of more than one energy should not be formed during decay. Also, the decay products should be stable.

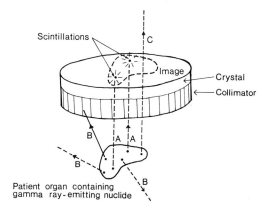

Fig. 5–1. Formation of an image in camera crystal by scintillations resulting from gamma ray absorptions. (A) Gamma rays used to construct image; (B) gamma rays that do not reach crystal; (C) gamma ray that passes through crystal without being absorbed. (From Rollo, F David (ed.): Nuclear Medicine Physics, Instrumentation and Agents. St. Louis, C.V. Mosby Co., 1977, p. 232, with permission.)

In addition to gamma photon energy, principal energy photons of high abundance should be formed during decay; radionuclides with more photons allow the administration of smaller activities without compromising image quality.

Some nuclear medicine studies are not performed with imaging devices and allow greater photon energy flexibility. Several procedures involve measurement of radioactivity in samples of blood or tissues using well-type detectors. With certain types of well detector systems, photon energies as low as 25 KeV and as high as several MeV can be adequately detected.

Decay Mode. Not all decay modes are useful in medicine. Alpha and beta decay, for instance, provide little, if any *diagnostic* benefit, since the particles they emit penetrate tissues for only very short distances and cannot be detected externally (the use of beta-emitting radionuclides for therapy is discussed in Chapter 17). Radionuclides that decay by β+ (positron) emission can be used for imaging, although the relatively high-energy 511 KeV photons produced by the positrons require the use of special imaging devices (called positron emission transmission tomography, or PETT, units). Generally, radionuclides that decay by isomeric transition (IT) or electron capture (EC) are preferred in medicine since these decay modes yield desirable gamma photons without the emission of beta particles.

Physical Half-Life. Each radionuclide decays with a definite physical half-life that is characteristic for a gamma radionuclide. The concept of physical half-life is discussed in Chapter 2. For clinical use, very short lived radionuclides may be impractical because of the expense and difficulties of daily air-freight shipments; very long lived radionuclides could also be undesirable since their use might result in unnecessary exposure of the patient to radiation.

Choice of Radionuclide. Presently, of more than 1400 known radionuclides, less than 50 have properties that make them suitable for use in humans. Table 5–1 lists the half-lives, modes of decay, and principal photon energies of radionuclides most widely used in nuclear medicine. Of these, Tc-99m offers nearly ideal properties for imaging. Although its 6.0-hour physical half-life might appear to limit its usefulness, the availability of the ^{99}Mo-^{99m}Tc generator facilitates its use almost anywhere in the world.

5.2 FACTORS AFFECTING BIOLOGICAL BEHAVIOR

Among the factors that significantly influence biodistribution (including rates of clearance from blood and other tissues) are the physical and chemical (physicochemical) states of radiopharmaceuticals. For example, substances soluble in blood that are also nonprotein-bound and have molecular weights of less than 5000 are usually rapidly excreted by the kidneys by glomerular filtration. Intravenously injected particulates, on the other hand, will be removed from blood by either the reticuloendothelial system (liver, spleen, and bone marrow) or the lungs, depending upon their size (Fig. 5–2). Additionally, radioactive gases such as Xe-133 or Kr-81m behave much like air and may be used to evaluate lung ventilation function. The classification in Table 5–2 describes the various physicochemical states of radiopharmaceuticals.

5.3 MECHANISMS OF LOCALIZATION

Specific patterns of radiopharmaceutical "uptake" can be described and conveni-

Table 5–1. Physical properties of selected radionuclides used in nuclear medicine's pharmacy.[t]

Radionuclide	Physical Half-life	Decay Mode	Principle Gamma Emission	Abundance (Emissions/100 disintegrations)
^{99m}Tc*	6.0 hr	IT	140 KeV	88
^{123}I	13.0 hr	EC	159 KeV	83
^{111}In	2.7 days	EC	173 KeV	89
			247 KeV	94
^{133}Xe	5.3 days	β⁻,γ	81 KeV	35
^{131}I	8.0 days	β⁻,γ	364 KeV	82

*Generator product formed from decay of ^{99}Mo (T$\frac{1}{2}$$_p$ = 67 hr).
[t]Although radioisotopes of carbon, hydrogen, nitrogen, and oxygen would appear obvious choices for use in medicine, their physical half-lives are either inappropriately short or very long.

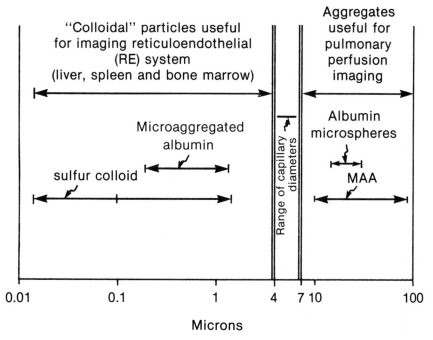

Fig. 5–2. Particles are removed from the bloodstream primarily by the reticuloendothelial (RE) system or by the lungs. This drawing allows the reader to compare the size ranges for different particulate radiopharmaceuticals that localize in either the lungs or the organs of the RE system. (Modified from Rhodes, BA, Croft, BY: Basics of Radiopharmacy. Saint Louis, C.V. Mosby, 1978.)

Table 5–2.   Classification system for physicochemical properties of radiopharmaceuticals and selected examples shown with individual clinical indications.

Physicochemical Type	Examples	Clinical Indication
1. Simple salts	^{123}I-sodium iodide	Thyroid imaging
	^{99m}Tc-sodium pertechnetate	Several—including brain, thyroid, salivary gland
2. Radioactive gases	^{127}Xe, ^{133}Xe, ^{81m}Kr	Pulmonary ventilation Cerebral blood flow
3. Particulates (colloids and aggregates)	^{99m}Tc-sulfur colloid	Liver imaging
	^{99m}Tc-macroaggregated albumin	Lung perfusion
4. Chelates of radiometals	^{99m}Tc-MDP	Skeletal imaging
	^{99m}Tc-DTPA	Renal imaging
	^{99m}Tc-disofenin	Hepatobiliary studies
5. Radiolabeled blood products	^{51}Cr-RBCs	Blood volume measurement
	^{99m}Tc-RBCs	Blood pool imaging
	^{111}In-WBCs	Abscess imaging
6. Radiolabeled analogs	^{75}Se-selenomethionine	Pancreas imaging
	^{11}C-valine	Pancreas imaging
	^{131}I-cholesterol (NP-59)	Adrenal imaging
	^{131}I-mIBG	Adrenal imaging
7. Radiolabeled antibodies	^{131}I-carcinoembryonic antibodies (CEA)	Tumor detection

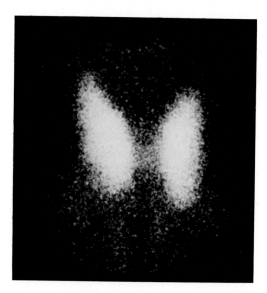

Fig. 5–3. Thyroid image obtained with ^{123}I-sodium iodide. This radiopharmaceutical is actively taken up by functioning cells of the thyroid gland.

ently grouped according to the types of *mechanisms of localization*. This term describes the tissue uptake pathways for radiopharmaceuticals and includes: (1) active transport, (2) simple diffusion, (3) capillary blockade, (4) phagocytosis, (5) cell sequestration, (6) compartmental localization, and (7) antigen-antibody complexation.

Active transport involves cellular metabolic processes that result in organ or tissue concentrations above plasma levels. Radioiodine, which is taken up by the thyroid gland, is the best-known example of a radiopharmaceutical that localizes by active transport. Measurement of the *amount* of radioiodine that concentrates in the thyroid gland ("thyroid uptake") provides a useful indication of thyroid function, while *scintiphotos* of radioiodine distribution in the thyroid can be used to evaluate gland size and shape, as well as the presence of thyroid nodules (Fig. 5–3).

Simple diffusion involves the movement of a substance from regions of higher concentration to regions of lower concentration. Diffusion of substances from plasma into the brain is controlled by a complex anatomic and physiologic mechanism known as the blood-brain barrier (BBB), which selectively limits the free exchange of substances between the blood and brain. Essential nutrients pass the BBB, as do certain lipid-soluble materials; however, most water-soluble substances (including many radiopharmaceuticals) are prevented from reaching normal, healthy brain cells. Pathologic conditions such as neoplasm, infarction, and inflammation result in "gaps" in the BBB, which permit diffusion of radiopharmaceuticals into affected tissues. Falling levels of the radiopharmaceutical in blood (resulting from rapid excretion of water-soluble radiopharmaceuticals by the kidneys) compared to the relatively constant amount in lesions permits visualization of the target tissue as areas of radiopharmaceutical uptake (Fig. 5–4).

Capillary blockade is based on the fact that upon intravenous injection, particles larger than red blood cells will become lodged in the first capillary bed they encounter. When radiolabeled particles of the appropriate size are injected intravenously, they lodge in the capillary bed of the lungs and depict lung blood supply. The particles occlude capillaries according to the vessel location within the organ and in proportion to the regional blood supply (Fig. 5–5). Thus, lung tissues with either a diminished or an absent blood supply, characteristic in chronic lung disease or pulmonary embolism, receive less blood and hence fewer radiolabeled particles than normally perfused lung tissues receive. Therefore, scintillation camera images would reveal these nonperfused areas as devoid of radioactivity. Although these particles can be considered microemboli, they do not represent a significant risk to the patient; they occlude only a small percentage of the existing capillaries and are composed of biodegradable materials.

Phagocytosis is the primary function of the cells of the reticuloendothelial (RE) system. The phagocytosis process involves recognition and removal of small foreign

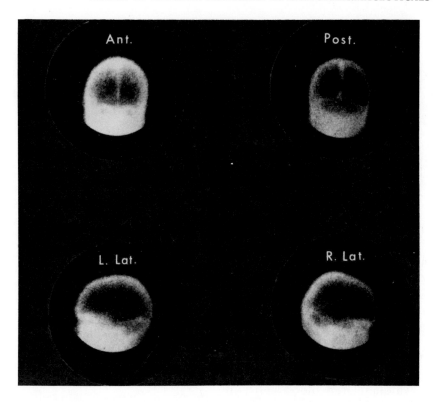

Fig. 5–4. Brain scintiphotos obtained 1 hour after administration of ^{99m}Tc-gluceptate. No evidence of disease involving the brain is noted. This radiopharmaceutical localizes in brain lesions whenever breakdown in the blood-brain barrier occurs.

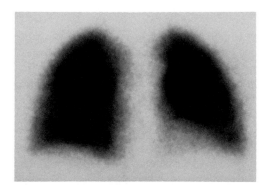

Fig. 5–5. Anterior image of normal, healthy lungs performed with ^{99m}Tc-macroaggregated albumin (MAA). Areas of lung with blood supply shown as "hot" (dark) areas. In lung disease, nonperfused areas would show as "cold" (gray or white) regions on scintillation image.

particles in the blood. The largest mass of RE cells is in the liver ($\cong$85%), with the remaining cells in the spleen ($\cong$10%) and bone marrow ($\cong$5%). When radioactive particles smaller than red blood cells are injected intravenously, they are recognized as foreign and rapidly removed from the blood by the RE cells. Since RE cells are distributed homogeneously in the liver and spleen, the uptake of radiolabeled colloid particles (such as ^{99m}Tc-sulfur colloid) by these organs permits, through scintillation imaging, observation of organ size, shape, and position (Fig. 5–6).

Cell sequestration is the process by which the spleen recognizes and removes damaged red blood cells and cells that are nearing the end of their life expectancy. In spleen sequestration studies, the patient's own red blood cells are withdrawn, radiolabeled, slightly damaged, and then

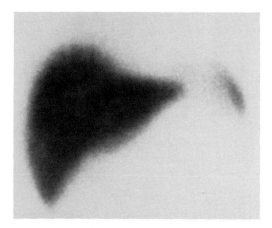

Fig. 5–6. Scintillation image of liver taken anteriorly of a patient injected with 99mTc-sulfur colloid.

reinjected. Because the damaged cells will be taken up only by the spleen, the spleen can be imaged without the interference of the liver, which would appear if a radiocolloid study were performed. Several different radiopharmaceuticals have been used to radiolabel red blood cells for splenic sequestration studies (Table 5–3).

Compartmental localization occurs when radiopharmaceuticals are introduced directly into well-defined body compartments and remain there long enough for imaging to be performed. For example, nondiffusible radiopharmaceuticals injected directly into the cerebral spinal fluid (CSF) space provide useful diagnostic information on CSF kinetics in patients with hydrocephalus or in patients suspected of having CSF rhinorrhea. Other applications of compartmental localization include

studies of gastrointestinal function, performed by timing the movement of orally administered insoluble radiopharmaceuticals through the GI tract, and lung ventilation studies, including administration of physiologically inert radioactive gases by inhalation.

Antigen-antibody complexation is a relatively new technique for tumor localization, although the principle of this method was demonstrated in animals as early as the 1950s. A variety of radiolabeled (usually I-131) antibodies to tumor-associated antigens have been investigated for potential usefulness in tumor detection. To date, most imaging studies using radiolabeled antibodies have been disappointing because of the low tumor specificity of the radiolabeled antibodies. This is most likely related to the polyclonal antibody source. Recently, the development of hybridization techniques for preparing highly specific monoclonal antibodies has stimulated interest in these substances for tumor imaging. One of the more successful radiolabeled antibodies for imaging has been "p97", an antimelanoma antibody investigated by Dr. Steve Larson at the National Institutes of Health (NIH). Tumor detection with radiolabeled antibodies is discussed in Chapter 13.

REFERENCES

1. Burns, HD: Design of radiopharmaceuticals. *In* The Chemistry of Radiopharmaceuticals. Edited by ND Heindel, HD Burns, T Honda, LW Brady. New York, Masson Publishing Company, 1978.
2. Counsell, RE, Ice, RD: The design of organ imaging radiopharmaceuticals. *In* Drug Design, Vol. 6. Edited by EJ Ariens. New York, Academic Press, 1975.
3. McAfee, JG, Subramanian, G: Agents for radioisotopic imaging. *In* Clinical Scintillation Scanning, 2nd Ed. Edited by L Freeman, PM Johnson. New York, Grune and Stratton, 1975.
4. Wagner, HN Jr, Emmons H: Characteristics of an ideal radiopharmaceutical. *In* Radioactive Radiopharmaceuticals. Edited by GA Andrews, KM Knisely, HN Wagner Jr. CONF-651111, National Technical Information Service, Springfield, Virginia, U.S. Department of Commerce, 1966.

Table 5–3. Radiopharmaceuticals employed for red blood cell labeling for splenic sequestration studies.

Agent	Physical T½	Cell Damaging Technique
51Cr-sodium chromate	27.8 days	Heat
99mTc-sodium pertechnetate (pretreatment with stannous ions)	6.0 hr	Heat

Radiation Dose and Risks

The increasing number of nuclear medicine procedures performed yearly results in the irradiation of larger numbers of humans by radioactive materials. The amount of radiation (i.e., the "dose") they receive from these internally localized radiopharmaceuticals is a measure of potential risk and must be weighed against the expected benefits of the procedure. Radiation dose and risk can only be estimated, however, because numerous factors produce uncertainties in radiation dose estimation, particularly when applied to specific patients. These include, in addition to fundamental nuclear properties, the chemical and physical states of the radionuclide (i.e., the radiopharmaceutical), the redistribution and elimination of radionuclides, the presence of disease states, and the patient's age.

6.1 RADIATION DOSE UNITS

Rad: The Unit of Absorbed Dose. Since biological effects relate to energy absorbed in the living system, the most important units refer to absorbed energy. The basic unit of radiation absorbed dose is the *rad*. It is a measure of the amount of energy absorbed per unit mass of the absorbing material, in this case tissue. Specifically, 1 rad is defined as equal to an energy deposition of 100 ergs per gram in the medium of interest.

Rem: The Dose Equivalent Unit. The *rem* was developed in response to a considerable body of evidence indicating that biological effects produced by some radiations such as alpha particles and neutrons are more damaging per rad than less densely ionizing radiations (such as x rays, gamma rays, and beta particles). To account for this difference, a factor called "dose equivalent" was introduced, the basic unit of which is the rem. The factor Q, or "quality factor," is a measure of the relationship of the effectiveness of a standard dose of x ray to the dose of another radiation required to produce the same effect. Thus,

$$\text{rems} = Q \times \text{rads}$$

For the x and gamma rays and the beta particles emitted by the radionuclides important in nuclear medicine, Q = 1, and rads and rems are essentially equivalent to each other. For neutrons and protons, Q = 10, and for alpha particles, Q = 20.

6.2 FACTORS THAT DETERMINE RADIATION DOSE

Amount of Radioactivity Administered. For any radionuclide, the dose of radiation to body organs and the total body is related directly to the amount of radioactivity administered. The greater this amount of activity, the greater the radiation dose.

Types of Radiation Emitted. Most procedures in nuclear medicine depend on the external detection of gamma rays that are emitted from inside the body; however, other emitted radiations may add to the radiation dose and yet yield no clinical benefit. In fact, most of the radiation dose from gamma-emitting radionuclides is due not to the gamma emissions but to beta particles, conversion electrons, and low-energy x rays emitted at the same time.

To reduce radiation dose, it is preferable to use radionuclides that emit gamma rays but lack beta particles and have few other associated low-energy radiations (Tc-99m is an example of such a radionuclide).

Physical Half-Life of the Radionuclide. Because most types of imaging equipment used in nuclear medicine have limited sensitivity, for some procedures there is no alternative to administering to the patient relatively large amounts of radioactivity. Large amounts of radioactivity can be administered and still have radiation dose levels within acceptable limits, if the radionuclide's physical half-life *is short*. This is true because the length of time the radioactivity remains in any organ is a primary factor affecting the radiation dose received by the organ. The trend, therefore, is toward the clinical use of radionuclides with shorter half-lives.

Chemical and Physical State. The biodistribution of a radiopharmaceutical and the radiation dose received by the patient are greatly affected by the chemical and physical form of the radionuclide. Consider as an example radiopharmaceuticals labeled with I-131, a radionuclide that in its simplest ionic state (as sodium iodide) is used to evaluate the thyroid gland. For example, the diagnostic utility of I-131 can be expanded beyond thyroid evaluation if this radionuclide is bound to tissue-specific compounds such as radioiodinated orthoiodohippuric acid, which is excreted by the kidneys, or ^{131}I-mIBG, a substrate that localizes in the adrenal glands. In these radiopharmaceuticals, however, any unbound ("free") I-131 is undesirable, since in its ionic state I-131 localizes in the thyroid, resulting in this gland's unnecessary exposure to radiation. Ideally, all of the radioactivity present in radiopharmaceuticals should be in the desired chemical form. Occasionally, it is advisable to ana-

lyze radiopharmaceuticals prior to patient administration in order to determine the amount of radioactivity that is present in the desired chemical form. This procedure, called testing for "tagging efficiency," involves analysis of radiochemical purity. The specific tests for radiochemical purity are discussed in Chapter 9.

Redistribution and Clearance of Radionuclides In nuclear medicine, radiopharmaceuticals are usually administered by intravenous injection and are rapidly distributed throughout the plasma volume and from plasma into other body "compartments." They may be concentrated for a time in one or more organs, but eventually they are eliminated by a combination of two processes: biological excretion and radioactive decay.

The rate of radiopharmaceutical clearance resulting from radioactive decay is indicated by the physical half-life (T_p) of the radionuclide. The rate of biological elimination of a radiopharmaceutical, known as the biological half-life (T_b) is rarely known with accuracy. Both processes decrease the amount of radioactivity in the body and combine to give what is called the "effective half-life" (T_e), a time less than either the physical or biological half-life.

$$T_e = T_p T_b/(T_p + T_b)$$

Unfortunately, data on biological elimination of most of the commonly used radiopharmaceuticals is scant, and elimination rates among normal individuals vary greatly. A further complication exists in that most individuals studied by procedures in nuclear medicine are ill, and these pathological states profoundly affect biological handling of radiopharmaceuticals. As a result, the effective half-life is difficult to estimate, despite its importance as a determinant of radiation dose.

Pathologic Conditions. Most available information on the distribution of internally administered radiopharmaceuticals does not take into consideration the effect of various illnesses, even though in prac-

Table 6–1.   Effect of liver disease on radiation dose from ^{99m}Tc-sulfur colloid.*

| Tissue | Normal Liver | Diffuse Parenchymal Disease | |
		Early Intermediate	Diffuse Intermediate
Liver	2.7	1.7	1.3
Spleen	1.7	2.2	3.4
Bone Marrow	0.22	0.36	0.63
Testes	0.0088	0.017	0.026
Ovaries	0.045	0.065	0.096
Whole Body	0.15	0.15	0.14

*Technical product data, Mallinckrodt, Inc.

tice it is the rule rather than the exception to have pathologic changes in the organ being studied. Under these circumstances, pathologic conditions can have profound effects upon radiopharmaceutical biodistribution. For example, approximately 85% of both ^{99m}Tc-sulfur colloid and ^{99m}Tc-microaggregated colloid is usually distributed in the liver, with the remainder divided between the spleen and bone marrow. In liver disease, however, only 60 to 70% of either radiopharmaceutical may concentrate in liver, while the remainder is shared between the spleen and bone marrow. In this situation, because the spleen is smaller than the liver, radiopharmaceutical concentration in the spleen may actually exceed that in the liver and result in a splenic radiation dose much higher than anticipated (Table 6–1).

Age of the Patient. Patient age and size can also affect radiation dose. Not only are organs of infants and children smaller than adults, but proportions are also different. For this reason, infants and children receive greater radiation doses than adults even if the amounts of radiopharmaceuticals administered are reduced according to

Table 6–2.   Four useful methods for the calculation of pediatric radiopharmaceutical dosages. Differences in calculation method involve the use of either age, weight, body mass or combinations thereof as primary considerations.

1. Clark's rule (weight)

$$\frac{\text{weight in lbs} \times \text{adult dose}}{150 \text{ lb}}$$

2. Webster's rule (age)

$$\frac{\text{age (in yrs)} + 1}{\text{age} + 7} \times \text{adult dose}$$

3. Young's rule (age)

$$\frac{\text{age (in yrs)}}{\text{age} + 12} \times \text{adult dose}$$

4. Body Surface Area^A

| Weight | | Surface Area (m²) | Fraction of Adult Dose* |
kg	lb		
2	4.4	0.15	0.09
4	8.8	0.25	0.14
6	13.2	0.33	0.19
8	17.6	0.40	0.23
10	22.0	0.46	0.27
15	33.0	0.63	0.36
20	44.0	0.83	0.48
25	55.0	0.95	0.55
30	66.0	1.08	0.62
35	77.0	1.20	0.69
40	88.0	1.30	0.75
45	99.0	1.40	0.81
50	110.0	1.51	0.87
55	121.0	1.58	0.91

*Based on average adult surface area of 1.73 m².
^{A}From Modell, W: Principles of the choice of drugs. *In* Drugs of Choice, 1958–1959. Edited by W Modell. St. Louis, C.V. Mosby, 1958.

body weight (see Appendix D for radiation dose estimates in children).

Several methods have been used to calculate pediatric dosages of radiopharmaceuticals (Table 6–2). In all situations, it is important to use the least amount of radioactivity that will allow the study to be performed effectively.

6.3 CALCULATION OF RADIATION DOSE ESTIMATES

MIRD Committee. In 1964, an ad hoc committee of the Society of Nuclear Medicine was formed to determine the absorbed dose to patients who were administered radiopharmaceuticals. Since that time, the Medical Internal Radiation Dose (MIRD) Committee has compiled tissue distribution data, radionuclide decay schemes, data on the fraction of energy absorbed for specific radionuclides in various organs of the body, and anatomic models for computing absorbed dose. These data are available as the MIRD Committee reports and pamphlets from the Society of Nuclear Medicine.

Calculation of Dose Rate. An introduction to the basic principles of calculating radiation dose must begin with an explanation of the relationship between dose rate and activity. If we have a large volume of soft tissue with a radioactive material mixed uniformly within, we almost intuitively know that the dose rate to the tissue varies directly with the concentration (activity per unit mass) and the amount of energy released per nuclear transformation.

The mathematical equation for dose ratio would be

$$\dot{D} = k \cdot \frac{A}{m} \cdot \bar{E}$$

$\dot{D}$ = the dose rate (rads/hr)
k = constant, which depends on the units used
A = the amount of activity (in microcuries) in the tissue volume

m = the time mass in grams (so A/m is the concentration)
$\bar{E}$ = the average energy released per transformation

Because MIRD has chosen to express $\dot{D}$ in rads per hour, A in microcuries, m in grams, and $\bar{E}$ in MeV per nuclear disintegration, the constant, k, becomes 2.13, and the previous equation is

$$\dot{D} = 2.13 \cdot \frac{A}{m} \cdot \bar{E}$$

In reality, a Δ value for energy emitted exists for each mode of decay, and, where more than one mode exists, each mode is weighted by n, the mean number per disintegration. Thus, the dose rate to tissue can be expressed as

$$\dot{D} = \frac{A}{m} (n_1\Delta_1 + n_2\Delta_2 + - - - -)$$

or

$$\dot{D} = \frac{A}{m} \Sigma n\Delta$$

where Σ symbolizes summation.

Absorbed Fraction. Each particle or photon has unique properties that determine its range in tissue. Charged particles have a short range, so their energy is absorbed close to their origin. Photons, on the other hand, can travel great distances before interacting, so they are less likely to be completely absorbed within the tissue volume. A correction factor (ϕ), the absorbed fraction, is used to correct for radiation not absorbed within the tissue volume. For nonpenetrating radiations such as beta particles, the fraction absorbed locally (ϕ) is 100%, or 1 if expressed as a fraction. For photons the value of ϕ is usually less than 1. Thus, the dose rate to the tissue volume would be

$$\dot{D} = \frac{A}{m} \Sigma n\Delta\phi$$

Average Life. As the atoms decay, the dose rate within the tissue volume decreases exponentially with time (related to the half-life) and approaches zero. If we assume *hypothetically* that the dose rate remains constant (does not decrease) at a rate equal to the initial dose rate, the same amount of energy (or dose) would be deposited in an amount of time equal to the average life (T_a), which is 1.44 times the physical half-life.

$$T_a = 1.44\ T_{1/2}$$

Cumulated Concentration. The instantaneous dose rate will decrease with time through decay and biological removal from the tissue volume (as given by the effective half-life, T_e). If A is the initial concentration in μCi we can use the concept of average life to determine the cumulated activity ($\tilde{A}$) as

$$\tilde{A} = 1.44 \cdot A \cdot T_e$$

where T_e is given in hours.

Organ Dose, Absorbed Fraction. The equation for calculation of the radiation dose to an organ from radiations emitted by decaying radionuclide in that organ is thus given by

$$\bar{D} = \frac{\tilde{A}}{m} \Sigma n \Delta \phi$$

Values of Δ are tabulated in MIRD Pamphlet 10, and MIRD Pamphlet 5 provides values of absorbed fraction for 16 source organs, 25 target organs, and 12 photon energies.

Even when values of $\tilde{A}$ are available, the calculation of dose can be a formidable and tedious task because of the necessity of finding each value of Δ and ϕ, then summing their products for each target-source combination. Because the sum of $\Delta \phi$ is uniquely specified, MIRD has developed the term *absorbed dose per unit cumulated activity (S).*

Organ Dose per Unit Cumulated Activity (S). Since the sum of the products of Δ and ϕ (designated $\Sigma \Delta \phi$) for each radionuclide has been uniquely specified, and the values of m, the mass of the organ, are ordinarily those for a standard phantom

man, it is convenient to introduce the quantity

$$S(r_k \leftarrow r_h) = \Sigma \frac{\Delta \phi}{m}(r_k \leftarrow r_h)$$

where r_k is the target organ and r_h is the source organ. Thus we can calculate dose with the simple formula

$$\bar{D}\ (r_k \leftarrow r_h) = \tilde{A}\ S(r_k \leftarrow r_h)$$

or

$$\bar{D} = \tilde{A}\ S$$

Since there are usually several source organs (r_h), the total average dose to the target organ r_k is given by the sum of the dose from each. Values of S for over 110 radionuclides are given in MIRD Pamphlet 11.

EXAMPLE

As an example, we will estimate the dose to the liver from 1 mCi of ^{99m}Tc-sulfur colloid.

Our assumptions will be:

85% uptake by the liver
7% uptake by the spleen
5% uptake by the bone marrow with instantaneous uptake
3% distributed in the remainder of the body

and $T_e = T_p$ for Tc-99m (6.0 hr).

The cumulated activities are calculated using

$$\tilde{A} = 1.44\ A\ T_e\ \mu\text{Ci-hr}$$

Thus for 1 mCi (1000 μCi) administered

$$\tilde{A}_{\text{LIV}} = 1.44 \times 0.85 \times 1,000 \times 6$$
$$= 7344$$

$$\tilde{A}_{\text{SPL}} = 1.44 \times 0.07 \times 1,000 \times 6$$
$$= 605$$

$$\tilde{A}_{\text{RBM}} = 1.44 \times 0.05 \times 1,000 \times 6$$
$$= 432$$

The total dose to the liver ($\bar{D}$ Li) would be calculated using the S values from Table 6–3

$$\bar{D}_{\text{LIV}} = \tilde{A}_{\text{LIV}} \cdot S\ (LIV \leftarrow LIV) + \tilde{A}_{\text{SPL}} \cdot S\ (LIV \leftarrow SPL)$$

$$+ \tilde{A}_{\text{RBM}} \cdot S\ (LIV \leftarrow RBM)$$

$$= 7344 \times 4.6 \times 10^{-5} + 605 \times 9.8 \times 10^{-7}$$

$$+ 432 \times 1.6 \times 10^{-6}$$

$$= 0.338 + 0.0006 + 0.0006$$

$$\bar{D}_{\text{LIV}} = 0.339\ \text{rads}$$

Table 6–3.   S values for sulfur colloid Tc-99m.

$(r_k \leftarrow r_h)$	S
(liver ← liver)	4.6E–05
(liver ← spleen)	9.8E–07
(liver ← marrow)	1.6E–06

(4.6E–05 means 4.6×10^{-5})
(From MIRD Pamphlet 10. Dillman, LT, Von der Lage, FC: Radionuclide decay schemes and nuclear parameters for use in radiation-dose estimation. New York, Society of Nuclear Medicine, 1975.)

6.4   RADIATION DOSE AND RADIOPHARMACEUTICALS

Radiopharmaceuticals used in the majority of diagnostic studies in adults ordinarily result in organ doses of less than 5 rads (Table 6–4), with doses to the whole body of less than 0.2 rads. Radiation doses below 10 rads are considered to be in the "low-dose" range.

6.5   TYPES OF RADIATION EFFECTS

The possible risks from radiation doses in the "low-dose" range are limited to those effects resulting from altered indi-

Table 6–4.   Radiation dose levels for diagnostic use of radiopharmaceuticals (the *organ* receiving the highest dose is indicated). Radiation dose levels are estimates using average activities administered to adults.

High Doses (>5 rads)
[131]I-sodium iodide for thyroid imaging (thyroid)
[131]I-iodocholesterol for adrenal imaging (adrenal)
[75]Se-Selenomethionine for pancreas imaging (liver)
^{99m}Tc-DMSA for renal imaging (kidney)

Medium (1–5 rads)
[99m]Tc-pertechnetate for brain imaging (thyroid)
^{99m}Tc-DTPA for brain imaging (bladder)
[99m]Tc-sulfur colloid for liver imaging (liver)
[99m]Tc-diphosphonates for bone imaging (bone)
[67]Ga-citrate for tumor and abscess imaging (large intestine)
[201]Tl-chloride for heart imaging (kidney)
[51]Cr-sodium chromate for red cell studies (spleen)
[99m]Tc-gluceptate for brain or kidney imaging (kidney)

Low (<1 rad)
[99m]Tc-red blood cells for blood pool imaging (blood)
^{99m}Tc-MAA for lung imaging (lung)
[131]I-hippuran for kidney function studies (kidney)
[127]Xe and ^{133}Xe for lung ventilation imaging (lung)

Additional radiation dose estimates for commonly used radiopharmaceuticals may be found in Appendix B.

vidual cells (damaged either singly or in small numbers) and include induction of cancer, genetic effects, and effects on an embryo. Effects such as cell depletion of bone marrow and impaired fertility or sterility have thresholds well above the radiation dose levels associated with diagnostic radiopharmaceuticals. In fact, based upon current knowledge, the potential risk of radiation effects related to the use of radiopharmaceuticals is low. The following discussion is offered, however, as a concise review of the hazards of radiation exposure and the relative risk of such effects from the use of radioactive materials as pharmaceuticals.

6.6   INDUCTION OF CANCER

It has been known for at least 70 years that exposure to ionizing radiation increases cancer incidence. In fact, more is probably known about the carcinogenic effects of ionizing radiation than about those of any other environmental carcinogen. The most significant human experience comes from the survivors of the 1945 Hiroshima and Nagasaki atomic bomb blasts, but there is other experience from medical and early occupational radiation exposure. These studies have produced information sufficient to state that cancer induction is probably the greatest risk to humans exposed to low levels of radiation. The major types of well-documented radiation-induced cancer in humans are breast, thyroid, and lung cancers, leukemia, and alimentary tract cancer (in order of decreasing risk).

Contrary to popular belief, exposure to high doses of radiation does not imply almost certain cancer induction. In fact, high doses (>100 rads) are *known* to cause only a small increase in the background cancer rate among exposed individuals. For example, studies of approximately 80,000 Japanese atomic bomb survivors matched against controls have shown (through

1978) only 250 excess deaths from leukemia and cancer in this heavily irradiated group.

Although the risks of various radiation-induced cancers *at high doses* are fairly well established, it is difficult to estimate precisely the risk at low doses because the risk is so low. This determination is further complicated by the difficulty in distinguishing radiation-induced cancers from the many spontaneous cancers, and by the long "latent period" (up to 40 years) between exposure and development of a cancer. The sample sizes required to demonstrate a small increase in cancer induction are impractically large; for example, if the higher incidence is proportional to the dose and if 1000 exposed and 1000 control subjects are required to test for cancer excess at 100 rads, then about 10 million would be required in each group for 1 rad. Thus, it may be *impossible* to observe such a risk of low-dose radiation *directly*.

Estimates of the risk of cancer induction are based on estimates of the increase in cancer observed in humans following exposure to higher (>100 rads) doses. The usual practice has been to assume a *linear* or proportional relationship between dose and effect, with no threshold. For example, if a dose of 100 rads given to 1000 people (100 × 1000 = 100,000 person-rads) produced 20 extra cancers, the same number of cancers, in this case 20, would be predicted from a dose of 1 rad given to 100,000 people (1 × 100,000 = 100,000 person-rads). Most experiments using the types of radiations emitted by radionuclides used in nuclear medicine indicate a less than proportional (curvilinear) response.

If the actual dose-response curve for radiation-induced cancers is curvilinear, then estimates made using the linear model would overestimate the risks of low doses. For this reason, estimates based upon the linear (proportional) mode are usually regarded by most scientists as an upper limit of risk.

The estimates of the risks of radiation exposure to humans in recent reports center around 100 lifetime fatal cancers (with an upper limit of about 200) induced by a dose of 1 rad in an exposed population of 1 million. When this risk is compared to the spontaneous lifetime risk of about 160,000 fatal cancers per million, two things are apparent: (1) the added cancer deaths would not be detectable (160,000 vs 160,100) and (2) the risk for an *individual* is very, very small.

There is currently *no evidence* that any *diagnostic* radionuclide test has produced cancer. The best evidence of the low risk can be seen in a recent report that measured the incidence of malignant thyroid tumors in 10,216 Swedish patients after exposure to diagnostic dosages of I-131 with a mean observation period of 17 years. The authors concluded that there was no elevation in the incidence of malignant thyroid tumors in the patients who had received I-131 when compared to figures for spontaneous tumors from the Swedish Cancer Registry.

6.7 GENETIC EFFECTS

About 10% of all liveborn humans will be seriously handicapped by genetic disorders at some time during their lifetimes. This high percentage makes the demonstration of radiation-induced genetic effects difficult, even at higher doses, because the mutations and chromosome aberrations produced by radiation are the same as those that occur spontaneously.

The estimation of genetic risk in humans is based largely upon animal studies, since there is *no significant* demonstration of radiation-induced gene mutation in humans. Even a study involving over 70,000 Japanese A-bomb survivors who became pregnant between 3 and 8 years after their exposure to radiation showed no indication in their offspring of any gross evidence of genetic damage such as malformations, stillbirths, or neonatal deaths. Current estimates are 5 to 75 additional serious genetic disorders per million liveborn per rem of parental radiation (the spontaneous level is 107,000 per million liveborn).

Thus the risk of a genetic defect in the child of a patient who had undergone a diagnostic test using radionuclides is insignificant compared to the spontaneous risk.

6.8 EFFECTS ON THE EMBRYO

There is little question that the developing embryo is highly sensitive to radiation. The major effects of high doses of radiation on the embryo are death, malformation, and reduced growth. These effects, since they relate to cell loss, are more likely to occur with increasing doses (with evidence for a "practical" threshold).

The stage of gestation during which the mother is irradiated is of major importance in determining effects, since the organ system that is differentiating at that time will be the most sensitive. During the period of organogenesis (about 11 to 50 days after fertilization), congenital malformation and retarded growth are the most likely consequences of radiation damage. Prior to this time (the preimplantation state) there is little chance of malformation, even at high radiation doses. Usually the embryo will either die or develop normally. After organogenesis (the fetal stage), growth retardation is the major effect from high doses.

Since there is scant evidence of any sort of an effect on the human embryo from doses less than 25 rads, NCRP Report 54 states that the risk of embryonic irradiation is "considered to be negligible at 5 rads or less when compared to the other risks of pregnancy, and the risk of malformation is significantly increased above control levels only at doses above 15 rad. Therefore, the exposure of the fetus to radiation arising from diagnostic procedures would rarely

Table 6–5. Conceptus dose estimates from radiopharmaceuticals.

Radiopharmaceutical	Conception Age (weeks)	Conceptus Organ	Dose Per Unit of Maternally Administered Activity (rad/mCi)
^{99m}Tc DTPA	1.5–6	Whole body	0.035
^{99m}Tc gluconate	1.5–6	Whole body	0.034
^{99m}Tc sodium pertechnetate	1.5–6	Whole body	0.037
^{99m}Tc polyphosphate	1.5–6	Whole body	0.025
^{99m}Tc sulfur colloid	1.5–6	Whole body	0.007
^{123}I sodium iodide	1.5–6	Whole body	0.032
^{131}I sodium iodide	1.5–6	Whole body	0.10
^{131}I sodium iodide	7–9	Whole body	0.88
^{131}I sodium iodide	11	Whole body	1.15
^{131}I sodium iodide	12–13	Whole body	1.58
^{131}I sodium iodide	20	Whole body	3.00
^{131}I sodium iodide	11	Thyroid	715
^{131}I sodium iodide	12–13	Thyroid	1338
^{131}I sodium iodide	20	Thyroid	5900
^{123}I sodium rose bengal	1.5–6	Whole body	0.13
^{131}I sodium rose bengal	1.5–6	Whole body	0.68
^{67}Ga citrate	1.5–6	Whole body	0.25
^{75}Selenomethionine	1.5–6	Whole body	3.8
^{59}Fe citrate	7–20	Whole body	38
^{59}Fe citrate	7–13	Liver	410
^{59}Fe citrate	20	Liver	330
^{59}Fe citrate	11	Spleen	61.2
^{59}Fe citrate	12–13	Spleen	140
^{59}Fe citrate	20	Spleen	186

(From Wagner, LK, Lester, RG, Saldena, LR: Exposure of the Pregnant Patient to Diagnostic Radiations. A Guide to Medical Management. Philadelphia, J.B. Lippincott Co., 1985, with permission.)

be cause, by itself, for terminating a pregnancy." For diagnostic procedures in nuclear medicine, the embryonic exposure is uniformly under 5 rads (Table 6–5).

An association between in utero exposure to diagnostic x rays and an increased risk of childhood leukemia and cancer has been established, but there still remains the question of whether there is a *causal* relationship.

6.9   LACTATION

The use of radiopharmaceuticals during lactation involves a risk that a breast-feeding child may receive radioactivity secreted in breast milk.

While a safe interval between administration of radioactivity and resumption of breast feeding has not been established for all radiopharmaceuticals, the following may be used as guidelines. For Tc-99m radiopharmaceuticals, breast feeding should be discontinued for 24 hours, and for I-123 labeled agents, resumption of breast feeding should not occur before 3 days. Breast feeding after the administration of longer-lived radiopharmaceuticals (e.g., I-131 and Ga-67) is generally contraindicated.

6.10   CONCLUSION

Radiopharmaceuticals are not used indiscriminantly; they are selectively employed as aids in the diagnosis or treatment of disease. For this reason, the benefits associated with the use of radiopharmaceuticals almost always outweigh any potential risks to *individual* patients.

REFERENCES

1. Bell, EG, McAfee, JG, Subramanian, G: Pediatric nuclear medicine. *In* Radiopharmaceuticals in Pediatrics. Edited by EA James, HN Wagner, Jr, RE Cooke. Philadelphia, W.B. Saunders Company, 1974.
2. Kato, H, Schull, WJ: Studies on the mortality of A-bomb survivors. 7. Mortality, 1950–1978: Part 1. Cancer mortality. Radiation Research, 90:395–432, 1982.
3. Kereiakas, JG, Rosenstein, M: Handbook of Radiation Doses in Nuclear Medicine and Diagnostic X-Ray. Boca Raton, Florida, CRS Press, 1980.
4. Kereiakas, JG, Thomas, SR, Gelfand, MJ, et al.: Dose evaluation in nuclear medicine. *In* Biological Risks of Medical Irradiations. Edited by GD Fullerton, DT Kapp, RG Waggener, EW Webster. American Association of Physicists in Medicine, Medical Physics Monograph No 5, New York, American Association of Physicists in Medicine, 1980, pp. 125–153.
5. Kieffer, CT, Suto, P: Management of the pediatric nuclear medicine patient (or children are not small adults). J Nucl Med Tech 11:13–17, 1983.
6. National Council on Radiation Protection and Measurements (NCRP), Report 54: Medical radiation exposure of pregnant and potentially pregnant women. Washington, D.C., 1977.
7. National Research Council, Advisory Committee on the Biological Effects of Ionizing Radiation (BEIR III): The effect on populations of exposure to low levels of ionizing radiation. Washington, D.C. National Academy of Science, 1980.
8. NCRP, No. 73. Protection in nuclear medicine and ultrasound diagnostic procedures in children. National Council on Radiation Protection and Measurements, Bethesda, Maryland, 1983.
9. Pizzarello, DJ, Witcofski, RL: Medical Radiation Biology. 2nd Ed. Philadelphia, Lea & Febiger, 1982.
10. Wagner, LK, Lester, RG, Saldana, LR: Exposure of the Pregnant Patient to Diagnostic Radiations. A Guide to Medical Management. Philadelphia, J.B. Lippincott Co., 1985.
11. Anderson, PO: Drugs and breast feeding. Drug Intell Clin Pharm. Vol 11. April, 1977, p. 217.
12. Ogunleye, OT: Assessment of radiation dose to infants from breast milk following the administration of ^{99m}Tc pertechnetate to nursing mothers. Health Phys 45:149–151, 1983.

The ^{99}Mo-^{99m}Tc Radionuclide Generator

Difficulties associated with the delivery and availability of short-lived radionuclides can be overcome through the use of radionuclide generators. These radionuclide supply systems make available desirable short-lived radionuclides (the "daughters") as they are formed by the decay of relatively longer-lived radionuclides (the "parents"). Central to this technique is an ion exchange column onto which a parent radionuclide is irreversibly bound. Because the daughter radionuclide is a different element it has no affinity for this column and can be separated when the proper solvent is used.

A variety of parent-daughter systems have been developed as radionuclide generators (Table 7–1). Among these the ^{99}Mo-^{99m}Tc generator is by far the most popular and serves as a prototype for the discussion of all other generator systems (Fig. 7–1).

7.1 THE ^{99}Mo-^{99m}Tc GENERATOR

The ^{99}Mo-^{99m}Tc generator system was developed in 1966 by Powell Richards at the Brookhaven National Laboratory. The characteristics of operation of the generator have remained almost unchanged from its original design. Aluminum trioxide ("alumina") is still used as the ion exchange material, and a vacuum-assisted process is employed for the removal and collection of the daughter radionuclide, Tc-99m.

This removal and collection process, in which the solvent (normal saline) is "pulled" over the column, is accomplished

by placing a sterile, pyrogen-free vacuum vial at the end opposite the saline source. The process of daughter removal is known as *elution*, the solvent used to collect the daughter is called the *eluant*, and the collected solution containing daughter Tc-99m is known as the generator *eluate*.

^{99}Mo-^{99m}Tc generators are either "wet-types" (WT) or "dry-types" (DT). A WT generator contains a reservoir of sterile eluant (i.e., normal saline) within the generator housing, while DT generators require that the eluant be placed on the generator for each elution. With the DT ^{99}Mo-^{99m}Tc generator, vials of sterile normal saline eluant are provided by the manufacturer, usually in volumes of 5 ml. Since the volume of normal saline eluant is uniform from one elution to the next, DT generators provide concentrations of activity that vary only with the amount of Tc-99m activity eluted. Since WT generators contain sufficient eluant to perform numerous elutions, the volume of eluate depends only upon the size of the vacuum vials employed. Commercial manufacturers of WT generators (Table 7–2) provide evacuated vials of different volumes (such as 5-, 10-, 20-, and 30-ml sizes) that enable the user to obtain relatively consistent activity concentrations over the usable lifetime of the generator.

7.2 PRODUCTION OF Mo-99

Mo-99 may be obtained either as a fission product of U-235 or from the neutron irradiation of stable Mo-98.

THE 99Mo-99mTc RADIONUCLIDE GENERATOR   55

Table 7-1.   Selected radionuclide generator systems for use in nuclear medicine.

Parent → Daughter	Parent				Daughter		
	$T\frac{1}{2}$ phys	Decay Mode	Principal Photon MeV	Production Method	$T\frac{1}{2}$ phys	Decay Mode	Photon MeV (%)
^{62}Zn → ^{62}Cu	9.2 hr	β⁺, EC	0.042(23) 0.51 (17) 0.59 (22)	^{63}Cu(p,2n)	9.8 min	β⁺	0.511(194)
^{68}Ge → ^{68}Ga	287 days	EC	—	^{66}Zn(^{4}He,2n)	68.3 min	β⁺, EC	0.511(178) 1.08 (3.5)
^{81}Rb → ^{81m}Kr	4.6 hr	β⁺, EC	0.446(23) 0.511(61)	^{79}Br(^{4}He,2n)	13 sec	IT	0.190(65)
^{99}Mo → ^{99m}Tc	67 hr	β⁻	0.181(7) 0.740(14) 0.780(5)	Fission, also ^{98}Mo(n,γ)	6.0 hr	IT	0.140(88)
^{113}Sn → ^{113m}In	115 days	EC	0.255(1.8)	^{112}Sn(n,γ)	1.66 hr	IT	0.392(62)
^{195m}Hg → ^{195m}Au	1.7 days	IT, EC	0.200(35) 0.261(32)	^{197}Au(p,2n)	30.6 sec	IT	0.261(68) 0.56(7.5)

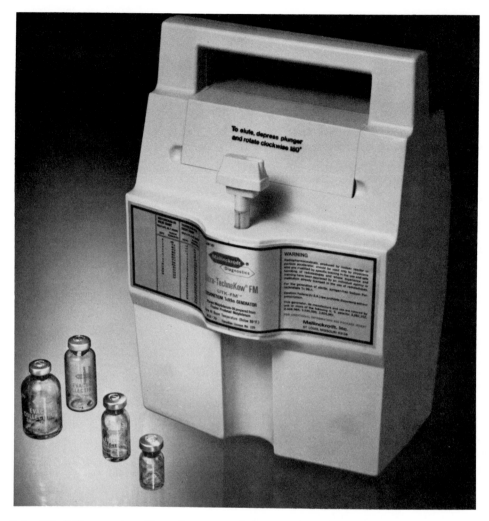

Fig. 7–1. ^{99}Mo-^{99m}Tc generator with sterile, evacuated elution vials. (Courtesy Mallinckrodt, Inc.)

Table 7–2.   Selected manufacturers of ^{99}Mo-^{99m}Tc generators according to basic design type (wet vs dry).

"Wet-type" (WT)
Mallinckrodt, Inc.
Medi-Physics, Inc.

"Dry-type" (DT)
E.R. Squibb & Sons
New England Nuclear

Fission product Mo-99 has several advantages in the manufacture of the ^{99}Mo-^{99m}Tc generators. Since it contains no carrier, has a high specific activity, and requires relatively small amounts of alumina to ensure complete binding, large amounts of fission product Mo-99 can be bound onto very small ion exchange columns. Thus, higher activity concentrations can be obtained.

Early ^{99}Mo-^{99m}Tc generators used Mo-99 prepared by both methods. Presently, only generators prepared from fission product Mo-99 are available in the U.S. Mo-99 is loaded onto alumina columns as molybdate (MoO_4^{-2}) in amounts ranging from a few hundred millicuries to several curies.

7.3   GROWTH KINETICS OF THE ^{99}Mo-^{99m}Tc GENERATOR

Following each elution, the amount of Tc-99m activity on the generator column

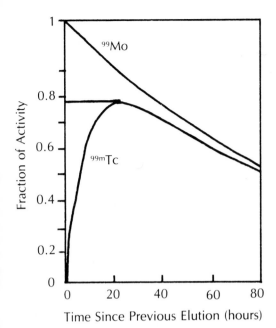

Fig. 7–2. Typical build-up and decay of Tc-99m from Mo-99. Following each generator elution, Tc-99m activity "grows-in" very rapidly, reaching maximum approximately 23 hours later. Following each elution, the growth curves are repeated.

"grows" or increases as a result of Mo-99 decay and reaches a maximum level approximately 23 hours later (Fig. 7–2). The kinetics of the growth curve demonstrate that Tc-99m activity, as a fraction of Mo-99 activity, continues to increase after this point, reaching transient equilibrium approximately 48 hours following elution. In the ^{99}Mo-^{99m}Tc generator, in which 86% of Mo-99 decays to Tc-99m (Fig. 7–3), the Tc-

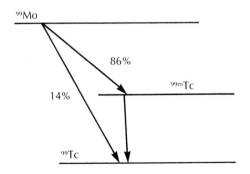

Fig. 7–3. Mo-99 decay scheme and the formation of Tc-99m.

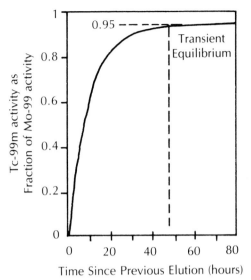

Fig. 7–4. Amount of Tc-99m activity on generator column as fraction of Mo-99 radioactivity. Transient equilibrium is demonstrated as technetium activity approaches constant fraction of molybdenum activity (0.946), approximately 48 hrs after previous elution.

99m activity on the generator column at transient equilibrium is equivalent to approximately 95% of Mo-99 activity (Fig. 7–4). For example, if at equilibrium the amount of Mo-99 activity is 1000 mCi, then approximately 950 mCi of Tc-99m is present.

7.4 CALCULATING GENERATOR YIELDS

In the daily preparation of Tc-99m radiopharmaceuticals it is often necessary to calculate the amount of Tc-99m activity that may be eluted from the ^{99}Mo-^{99m}Tc generator. This is accomplished by using basic decay equations, which determine the amount of Tc-99m formed from the decay of Mo-99 at any given time. Simply, this can be determined by answering these questions:

1. How much Mo-99 activity is present on the generator column?
2. How much Tc-99m activity has formed by Mo-99 decay at any given time?

3. What fraction of available Tc-99m is removed (the efficiency of elution)?

All Tc-99m generators are calibrated and labeled to show the amount of Mo-99 activity contained in the generator at a time usually within 24 hours of shipment from the manufacturer. Therefore, the first question (how much Mo-99 activity is present?) can be answered by using the calibration information and the standard decay equation

$$A = A_0 e^{-\lambda t}$$

where A_0 = Mo-99 activity on generator column at time of calibration
t = time elapsed since calibration

or by using decay tables such as that shown in Table 7–3.

The second question (how much Tc-99m activity is present on the column at any given time?) is somewhat more complex since it involves the decay rates for both Mo-99 and Tc-99m. The decay equation for the relationship of parent and daughter radionuclides is shown below.

A_1 = parent activity, λ_1 = parent decay constant
A_2 = daughter activity, λ_2 = daughter decay constant

$$\frac{A_2}{A_1} = \frac{0.86\,\lambda_2(e^{-\lambda_1 t} - e^{-\lambda_2 t})}{(\lambda_2 - \lambda_1)\,(e^{-\lambda_1 t})}$$

The factor of 0.86 is included in the decay equations because only 86% of Mo-99 atoms decays directly to Tc-99m.

Table 7–4 shows the calculated activity of Tc-99m on the generator column as a fraction of Mo-99 radioactivity.

Although the amount of Tc-99m activity present on a generator column at a given time can be calculated, it should not be assumed this entire activity will be eluted. Most generators, however, achieve an elution efficiency of approximately 80%.

SAMPLE PROBLEMS

Problem I

A ^{99}Mo-^{99m}Tc generator arrives at the nuclear pharmacy on Monday at 6:00 A.M. and is labeled to have contained 2200 mCi Mo-99 as of 6:00 A.M. on the previous Friday. If the generator is eluted immediately upon arrival, what is the minimum expected Tc-99m activity to be eluted?

Table 7–3. Mo-99 decay factors.

% activity remaining = orginal activity × decay factor
(decay factor = $e^{-\lambda t}$)

Time (t) (hr)	Decay Factor	Time (t) (hr)	Decay Factor	Time (t) (hr)	Decay Factor
−168	5.76	−48	1.65	36	0.687
−144	4.49	−44	1.58	40	0.659
−124	3.64	−40	1.52	44	0.632
−120	3.49	−36	1.46	48	0.606
−116	3.35	−32	1.40	52	0.581
−112	3.22	−28	1.34	56	0.558
−108	3.08	−24	1.28	60	0.535
−104	2.96	−20	1.23	64	0.513
−100	2.84	−16	1.18	68	0.492
−96	2.72	−12	1.13	72	0.472
−92	2.61	−8	1.09	96	0.368
−88	2.50	−4	1.04	120	0.286
−84	2.40	0	1.00	144	0.223
−80	2.30	4	0.959	168	0.174
−76	2.21	8	0.920	192	0.135
−72	2.12	12	0.882	216	0.105
−68	2.03	16	0.846	240	0.082
−64	1.95	20	0.812	264	0.064
−60	1.87	24	0.779	288	0.050
−56	1.79	28	0.747	312	0.039
−32	1.72	32	0.716	336	0.030

Table 7–4. Amounts of Tc-99m present on generator column at time (t) post generator elution and expressed as fraction of present Mo-99 radioactivity.

Fraction Tc-99m radioactivity (as compared to Mo-99 radioactivity)

$$= \frac{A_2}{A_1} = \frac{0.860\,\lambda_2(e^{-\lambda_1 t} - e^{-\lambda_2 t})}{(\lambda_2 - \lambda_1)\,(e^{-\lambda_1 t})}$$

Time (t) (hr)	$\frac{A_2}{A_1}$	Time (t) (hr)	$\frac{A_2}{A_1}$	Time (t) (hr)	$\frac{A_2}{A_1}$
0.5	0.048	10.0	0.614	27	0.890
1.0	0.094	10.5	0.631	28	0.896
1.5	0.138	11.0	0.647	29	0.901
2.0	0.179	11.5	0.662	30	0.905
2.5	0.218	12.0	0.677	32	0.913
3.0	0.255	13.0	0.704	34	0.919
3.5	0.290	14.0	0.728	36	0.924
4.0	0.324	15.0	0.750	38	0.929
4.5	0.356	16.0	0.769	40	0.932
5.0	0.386	17.0	0.787	44	0.937
5.5	0.414	18.0	0.803	48	0.940
6.0	0.441	19.0	0.817	54	0.943
6.5	0.467	20.0	0.830	60	0.944
7.0	0.492	21.0	0.841	66	0.945
7.5	0.515	22.0	0.852	72	0.946
8.0	0.537	23.0	0.861	78	0.946
8.5	0.558	24.0	0.870	84	0.946
9.0	0.578	25.0	0.877	90	0.946
9.5	0.596	26.0	0.884	96	0.946

Solution. In order to solve this problem, it is necessary to first determine the amount of Mo-99 present Monday at 6:00 A.M. on the generator column (Step One), then calculate the amount of Tc-99m that is also present (Step Two).

Step One. From Table 7–3, the 3-day decay factor (from Friday until Monday) for Mo-99 is 0.472. Therefore, the Mo-99 activity contained in this generator on Monday at 6:00 A.M. is:

generator calibration (Friday)	3-day post calibration factor Mo-99
2200 mCi Mo-99	× 0.472

Mo-99 activity on Monday

= 1038 mCi Mo-99

Step Two. Since the generator has not been eluted in the previous 72 hours, the generator has reached transient equilibrium (that is, the decaying parent forms daughter atoms at a rate that is proportional to the decay of the daughter atoms). From Table 7–4, the build-up fraction for Tc-99m as a fraction of Mo-99 activity at equilibrium is 0.946. Therefore, the Tc-99m activity available on the generator column is:

Mo-99 activity present on column	build-up factor for 72 hours	
1038 mCi Mo-99 ×	0.946	= 982 mCi Tc-99m

Answer. Since a generator elution efficiency of at least 80% is usually obtained, the amount of Tc-99m activity on the generator column must be reduced to 80% in order to determine the approximate Tc-99m activity that will be recovered in the generator elution. Therefore,

$$\frac{\text{Tc-99m activity}}{\text{on generator}} \times .80 = \frac{\text{expected minimum}}{\text{yield}}$$
$$982 \text{ mCi Tc99m} \qquad \boxed{786 \text{ mCi Tc-99m}}$$

Problem II

This same generator is next eluted the following morning (Tuesday) at 6:00 A.M. What is the expected Tc-99m yield?

Solution. Once again, it is necessary to determine first the amount of Mo-99 present (Step One), and then to calculate the Tc-99m activity (Step Two) in order to calculate the expected minimum yield of Tc-99m.

Step One. The amount of Mo-99 present on Tuesday can be determined by multiplying the previous day's activity (1038 mCi) by the 24-hour decay factor for Mo-99 (from Table 7–3). This value is 0.780.

$$\frac{\text{Monday's activity}}{} \qquad \frac{\text{24-hour}}{\text{decay factor}}$$

$$1038 \text{ mCi Mo-99} \times \quad 0.780 \quad = 810 \text{ mCi Mo-99}$$

Step Two. Because the time elapsed since the previous elution is only 24 hours, Tc-99m activity has built up to a level equivalent to 0.870. This build-up factor, taken from Table 7–4, expresses Tc-99m activity as a fraction of Mo-99m activity. Therefore,

$$\frac{\text{Mo-99 activity}}{} \quad \frac{\text{build-up}}{\text{factor}} \quad \frac{\text{Tc-99m activity on}}{\text{column}}$$

$$810 \text{ mCi} \qquad \times 0.870 \quad = 704 \text{ mCi Tc-99m}$$

Answer. Since the assumed elution efficiency is not less than 80%, the expected minimum yield is calculated as follows:

$$\frac{\text{Tc-99m activity}}{\text{on column}} \times .80 = \frac{\text{expected minimum}}{\text{yield}}$$
$$704 \text{ mCi} \qquad \boxed{564 \text{ mCi Tc-99m}}$$

All of the foregoing should not be taken to indicate that the ^{99}Mo-^{99m}Tc generator can be eluted only once daily. In fact, soon after each generator elution the rate of formation of daughter Tc-99m atoms is very high, after which the rate slows, eventually reaching equilibrium (Fig. 7–2). Table 7–4 shows that at 5 hours after elution nearly 40% of the maximum amount of Tc-99m activity can be obtained by a second elution, while the amount of Tc-99m in the next morning's elution (performed after

only a 19-hour build-up instead of a 24-hour build-up) would be decreased by less than 6% (81.7% vs 87.7%). Therefore, it is possible to perform a second or even a third elution of the ^{99}Mo-^{99m}Tc generator and not appreciably affect the next morning's Tc-99m yield.

7.5   FACTORS THAT DECREASE Tc-99m YIELD

Occasionally during elution of the ^{99}Mo-^{99m}Tc generator, Tc-99m may not be eluted but instead may remain absorbed on the column for two major reasons.

First, Tc-99m is eluted from the generator column only as the +7 state (pertechnetate); reduced Tc-99m species usually remain bound onto the alumina column. These reduced species can be created by reducing agents that may be formed by the radiolytic decomposition of water. This radiation-induced reaction is more likely on columns that contain very large activities. When radiolysis is suspected as a cause of low Tc-99m yield, the generator should be left undisturbed following elution for approximately 10 to 15 minutes, then re-eluted. This short time permits oxidation of reduced Tc-99m back to pertechnetate, which can be recovered during the next elution.

Secondly, poor Tc-99m yields can result from "channeling," a physical problem in which only a fraction of the column is accessible to the eluant. In this situation, significant Tc-99m (as pertechnetate) remains on the column. Usually, an "air pocket" in the column is responsible for the difficulty; with several repeated elutions the air pocket will disperse and the expected Tc-99m yield will be obtained with a subsequent elution.

7.6   HANDLING AND ASSAY OF GENERATOR ELUATE

Safe handling of the generator eluate is critical because it is usually the largest source of radioactivity in the nuclear pharmacy. During generator elution and at all times thereafter, the evacuated collection vial containing the generator eluate should be shielded and handled carefully.

Assay for Mo-99. Because Mo-99 is usually tightly bound to the alumina column, only minute quantities of Mo-99 normally appear in the generator eluate. The presence of Mo-99 in generator eluate is known as "moly breakthrough," and strict limits have been established for allowable quantities of Mo-99 (and other radionuclide contaminants) in generator eluate. ^{99}Mo administered to patients in generator eluate is taken up by the parenchymal cells of the liver and subjects that organ to a radiation dose of approximately 0.03 rads/μCi.

In the early days of the ^{99}Mo-^{99m}Tc generator, "moly breakthrough" occurred more frequently than it does today. Regardless, each generator eluate must be assayed for Mo-99 content. Mo-99 assay methods are discussed in Chapter 9.

7.7 OTHER RADIONUCLIDE GENERATOR SYSTEMS

Although the ^{99}Mo-^{99m}Tc generator is the most widely used, other radionuclide generators are available and are useful in certain clinical situations. Some of the more important radionuclide generator systems and their clinical uses are briefly discussed.

^{113}Sn-^{113m}In Generator. The very long physical half-life of Sn-113 (115 days) makes this generator particularly useful in those areas of the world where routine deliveries of the ^{99}Mo-^{99m}Tc generator might not be possible. The daughter, In-113m, has a 100-minute half-life and a principal emission of 393 KeV (64% yield); it decays by isomeric transition. Although the 393 KeV emission may be considered high energy (compared to the 140 KeV emission of Tc-99m), it can be adequately imaged with the scintillation camera.

^{68}Ge-^{68}Ga Generator. Positron-emitting Ga-68 (T½ = 68 minutes) is formed by the decay of Ge-68 (T½ = 280 days). Ga-68 is eluted from the generator as ^{68}Ga-EDTA and in this form has been used for brain imaging. Since Ga-68 is a positron-emitting radionuclide, its use is limited primarily to institutions with positron emission transmission tomography (PETT) imaging systems.

^{81}Rb-^{81m}Kr Generator. Ultra–short-lived Kr-81m (13 seconds) is produced from the decay of Rb-81 (T½ = 4.7 hr). The 190 KeV photons of Kr-81m are well suited for use with the scintillation camera. Kr-81m can be eluted from the generator with humidified oxygen or aqueous solutions. It is used primarily in the study of lung ventilation function. It may also be used to measure blood flow in various tissues and organs.

^{195m}Hg-^{195m}Au Generator. Au-195m is an ultra–short-lived radionuclide (30.6 seconds) useful for evaluating myocardial function by quantifying blood flow via the first pass technique. The high count rate from this rapidly decaying radionuclide requires the use of special camera systems (such as the multicrystal types) to generate adequate counting statistics.

REFERENCES

1. Hnatowich, DJ: A review of radiopharmaceutical development with short-lived generator-produced radionuclides other than ^{99m}Tc. Int J Appl Rad Isotop 28:169–181, 1977.
2. Lamson, M III, Hotte, CE, Ice, RD, et al: Practical generator kinetics. J Nucl Med Tech 4:21–27, 1976.
3. Lebowitz, E, Richards, P: Radionuclide generator systems. Semin Nucl Med 4:257–268, 1974.
4. Molinski, VJ: A review of ^{99m}Tc generator technology. Int J Appl Radiat Isot 33:811–819, 1982.
5. Richards, P: The technetium-99m generator. In Radioactive Pharmaceuticals. Edited by GA Andrews, RM Knisely, HN Wagner Jr. CONF-651111, National Technical Service, Springfield, VA, US Department of Commerce, 1966, pp. 323–334.
6. Steigman, J: Chemistry of the alumina column. Int J Appl Radiat Isot 33:829–834, 1982.
7. Yano, Y: Radionuclide generators: Current and future applications in nuclear medicine. In Radiopharmaceuticals. Edited by G Subramanian, BA Rhodes, JF Cooper, VJ Sodd. New York, Society of Nuclear Medicine, 1975, pp. 236–245.

Methods of Radiolabeling and Preparing Radiopharmaceuticals

Tc-99m eluted directly from the ^{99}Mo-^{99m}Tc generator as sodium pertechnetate can be used for several nuclear medicine procedures, including brain and thyroid imaging, organ blood flow imaging, and the labeling of red blood cells. While there are limitations to the clinical applications of ^{99m}Tc-sodium pertechnetate, its usefulness can be extended by complexing (or radiolabeling) this radionuclide onto a variety of tissue-specific compounds, thus forming several useful radiopharmaceuticals (Table 8–1).

Tc-99m will not label all compounds potentially useful in medicine. For this reason, other gamma-emitting radionuclides, such as radioisotopes of iodine, and transition metals, such as indium, must be used in preparing certain radiopharmaceuticals.

This chapter deals with processes for radiolabeling Tc-99m radiopharmaceuticals and selected non-Tc-99m agents.

8.1 PREPARATION OF Tc-99m AGENTS

Generator-produced ^{99m}Tc-sodium pertechnetate contains technetium in the chemically nonreactive +7 oxidation state and will not label compounds by simple addition. In fact, ^{99m}Tc-sulfur colloid is believed to be the only ^{99m}Tc radiopharmaceutical (besides ^{99m}Tc-sodium pertechnetate) that incorporates Tc-99m in the +7 oxidation state. The preparation of all other radiopharmaceuticals requires Tc-99m reduction to a chemically reactive species, generally the +4 oxidation state, in order for radiolabeling to occur.

^{99m}Tc-Sulfur Colloid. This radiopharmaceutical is prepared from commercially available kits that contain acid (either phosphorous or hydrochloric), sodium thiosulfate, a buffer, and gelatin. In the preparation of ^{99m}Tc-sulfur colloid, generator-produced ^{99m}Tc-pertechnetate is added to an acidic solution of sodium thiosulfate, and this mixture is heated in a boiling water bath for approximately 5 to 10 minutes. Following heating, the vial is briefly vented and a buffer is added to the mixture to neutralize pH (certain formulations may require an additional boiling of 5 to 8 minutes).

It is known that sodium thiosulfate reacts with acid to form elemental sulfur and sulfur dioxide, as shown below:

$$S_2O_3^{-2} + 2H^+ \rightarrow \downarrow S + SO_2 + H_2O$$

In the preparation of ^{99m}Tc-sulfur colloid, it is likely that the elemental sulfur condenses to form colloidal-size particles that in turn coprecipitate Tc-99m, probably as the heptasulfide (Tc_2S_7).

$$16\,H^+ + 2\,TcO_4^- + 7\,S^{-2} \rightarrow \downarrow Tc_2S_7 + 8\,H_2O$$

The particle size of ^{99m}Tc-sulfur colloid is 0.05 to 3.0 μ. Gelatin is used in most formulations as a stabilizer to prevent colloid particles from becoming undesirably large,

Table 8–1. USAN for radiopharmaceuticals containing Tc-99m.

Listed here are the U.S. Adopted Names (USAN) for the Tc-99m agents produced from the kits currently available. These USAN names are used in reporting the clinical use of the respective active agents.

The Food and Drug Administration has determined that the name of the nonradioactive kit shall be the name of the active agent produced by use of the kit (and known by the USAN given in the first column of the following table), preceded by the words "Kit for the preparation of." Thus, "Technetium Tc-99m albumin aggregated" is produced by the reaction of sodium pertechnetate Tc-99m with the ingredients of a kit labeled "Kit for the preparation of Technetium Tc-99m albumin aggregated."

In addition, clinical indications are shown in parentheses under the USAN for the active agent.

USAN for the Active Agent Produced from the Kit (clinical indication in parentheses)	Trademark for Kit	Manufacturer
Technetium Tc-99m albumin (blood pool imaging)	HSA	Medi-Physics
Technetium Tc-99m albumin aggregated (pulmonary perfusion)	AN-MAA	Syncor International
	TechneScan MAA	Mallinckrodt
	Pulmolite	Dupont-NEN
	Macrotec	Squibb
	MAA	Medi-Physics
Technetium Tc-99m albumin colloid (liver and spleen imaging)	Microlite	Dupont-NEN
	Microloid	Squibb
Technetium Tc-99m antimony trisulfide colloid (lymphoscintigraphy)	LymphoScan	Cadema
Technetium Tc-99m disofenin (hepatobiliary imaging)	Hepatolite	Dupont-NEN
Technetium Tc-99m gluceptate (brain and renal imaging)	AN-Glucotec	Syncor International
	Glucoscan	Dupont-NEN
Technetium Tc-99m mebrofenin (hepatobiliary imaging)	Choletec	Squibb
Technetium Tc-99m medronate (skeletal imaging)	AN-MDP	Syncor International
	MPI MDP Kit	Medi-Physics
	Osteolite	Dupont-NEN
	MDP-SQUIBB	Squibb
Technetium Tc-99m medronate disodium (skeletal imaging)	Amerscan MDP	Amersham
Technetium Tc-99m oxidronate (skeletal imaging)	Osteoscan-HDP	Mallinckrodt
Technetium Tc-99m pentetate (brain and renal imaging)	AN-DTPA	Syncor International
	DTPA	Medi-Physics
	MPI DTPA Kit	Medi-Physics
	Techneplex	Squibb
Technetium Tc-99m pyrophosphate (skeletal and myocardial infarction imaging)	AN-Pyrotec	Syncor International
	Sodium Pyrophosphate Kit	CIS Radiopharmaceuticals
	TechneScan PYP Kit	Mallinckrodt
	Phosphotec	Squibb
Technetium Tc-99m (Pyro- and trimeta-) phosphates (skeletal imaging)	Pyrolite	Dupont-NEN
Technetium Tc-99m succimer (renal imaging)	MPI DMSA Kidney Reagent	Medi-Physics
Technetium Tc-99m sulfur colloid (liver and spleen imaging)	TechneColl	Mallinckrodt
	Tesuloid	Squibb
	TSC Kit	Medi-Physics

(Table modified from USAN 1986: USAN and the USP Dictionary of Drug Names. The United States Pharmacopeial Convention, Inc. Easton, PA, Mack Printing Co., 1985. Permission granted.)

thus being trapped in the lungs (by capillary blockade) before reaching the liver. Factors that cause ^{99m}Tc-sulfur colloid particles to become undesirably large include excessive heating during preparation and the presence of high levels of Al^{+3} ions in the generator eluate used to prepare ^{99m}Tc-sulfur colloid. Aluminum ions bring about this effect by decreasing the normal repulsive electronegative colloidal surface charge (which stabilizes colloidal particle size), thus allowing colloidal aggregation. To prevent aggregation many sulfur colloid formulations contain EDTA, a chelating

1. Sodium borohydride
2. Stannous ions in acidic media
3. Electrolysis
4. Ferrous (II) ions with ascorbic acid

substance, which binds Al^{+3} ions. The test for Al^{+3} ions in ^{99}Mo-^{99m}Tc generator eluate is discussed in Chapter 9.

Reduced Tc-99m Radiopharmaceuticals. Other Tc-99m radiopharmaceuticals utilize reduced states of Tc-99m for labeling and are prepared using "kits." These products are commercially available as sterile, apyrogenic vials that contain a reducing agent, the compound to be labeled, and additional substances that facilitate the labeling reaction or enhance the stability of the formed Tc-99m complex.

Technetium can be reduced by several processes (Table 8–2). In practice, however, stannous ion reduction is preferred for its simplicity and effectiveness. This reduction method is used in the "kit-type" radiolabeling of most Tc-99m radiopharmaceuticals.

Since no stable isotope of technetium exists, it is difficult to determine (based upon nanomolar quantities of Tc-99m) the precise behavior of reduced technetium in binding reactions. In fact, much of the information regarding technetium chemistry is derived from what is known about other members of the same periodic group (Rh, Mn). It is generally accepted, however, that stannous reduction of technetium occurs in the manner shown below:

$$Sn^{+2} \rightarrow Sn^{+4} + 2 e^-$$
$$\text{Stannous} \quad \text{Stannic}$$
$$\text{ion} \quad \text{ion}$$

$$^{99m}TcO_4^- + 8 H^+ + 3 e^- \leftrightarrows {}^{99m}Tc \text{ (IV)} + 4 H_2O$$

Balancing these two equations yields the following composite reaction:

$$2 \, {}^{99m}TcO_4^- + 16 H^+ + 3 Sn^{+2} \leftrightarrows 2 \, {}^{99m}Tc \text{ (IV)} + 3 Sn^{+4} + 8 H_2O$$

In the presence of suitable compounds (usually chelates and some albumin partic-

ulates), reduced technetium will bind and form a radiolabeled complex (i.e., the radiopharmaceutical).

$$\underset{\text{Tc-99m}}{\text{Reduced}} + \underset{\text{Substance}}{\text{Chelating}} \leftrightarrows \underset{\text{Radiopharmaceutical}}{\text{Tc-99m (IV)}}$$

Usually, all that is required for the preparation of most Tc-99m radiopharmaceuticals (including sulfur colloid) is the addition to a specific kit of the desired activity and volume of generator-produced ^{99m}Tc-sodium pertechnetate. While the preparation of certain Tc-99m radiopharmaceuticals may require brief incubation periods or special procedures (e.g., ultrasonication or heating for brief periods) to ensure complete labeling, most kit-type radiopharmaceuticals may be prepared at room temperature and are ready for use only a few minutes after the addition of ^{99m}Tc-sodium pertechnetate.

Since few ($<10^{-9}$M) Tc-99m atoms are present in generator eluate, only a small amount of Sn^{+2} is required to ensure complete reduction. Although generally the amount of Sn^{+2} present in most kit formulations results in Sn^{+2}/Tc-99m ratios as large as 10^6, these amounts of tin are far below toxic levels.

Since the reduction of Tc-99m is reversible and reoxidation of reduced technetium back to pertechnetate may occur, kits are formulated to contain an excess of chelating agent in order to ensure complete binding of Tc-99m (IV).

8.2 REQUIREMENTS FOR LABELING WITH Tc-99m

While Tc-99m has near-ideal imaging properties, its chemistry, even when Tc-

Table 8–3.   Hydrophilic chemical groups useful for binding reduced technetium.

–OH	–NH$_2$
–COOH	–SOOH
–C=O	–SOONH$_2$
–PO$_4$	–OCH$_3$
–P$_2$O$_7$	

99m is in the chemically active reduced states, does not permit the radiolabeling for all types of radiopharmaceuticals. In fact, only compounds that possess hydrophilic groups (Table 8–3) bind the reduced Tc-99m species. Compounds containing only lipophilic groups will not bind technetium. Further, since technetium reduction by the stannous ion method occurs in acidic media, only compounds stable under these conditions may be radiolabeled with Tc-99m. Unfortunately, many biological compounds and a significant number of drug products are predominantly lipid soluble or unstable at acid pH and cannot be successfully radiolabeled with Tc-99m. Other radionuclides used to radiolabel such compounds are discussed later in this chapter.

8.3   FORMATION OF UNDESIRABLE Tc-99m COMPLEXES DURING RADIOLABELING

The apparent simplicity of the Tc-99m reduction and labeling process is actually deceiving, because several factors can affect Tc-99m labeling efficiency* and result in the presence of undesirable Tc-99m complexes. The causes and significance of the two primary Tc-99m impurities—unbound (free) pertechnetate and hydrolyzed, reduced technetium—are discussed below.

Unbound (Free) Pertechnetate. Oxygen or oxidizing agents can cause the reoxidation of reduced Tc-99m to pertechnetate. For this reason, normal saline solutions used either as the eluant or during kit prep-

aration should be free of oxidizing substances. As a preventive measure for oxidative effects, most kits are manufactured as lyophilized products, and air spaces in the vial are filled with an inert gas such as nitrogen. Even with these measures the inadvertent contamination of vials with room air (and oxygen) during the withdrawal of multiple doses can cause deterioration of the radiolabeled complex. To prevent destructive oxidative effects upon radiopharmaceuticals, some manufacturers have added antioxidants such as sodium ascorbate or gentisic acid.

Hydrolyzed, Reduced Tc-99m (HR-Tc). Reduced Tc-99m might also undergo hydrolysis in aqueous solution to form various insoluble hydrolysis products. Collectively, these radiocontaminants, called "hydrolyzed, reduced Tc-99m" (HR-Tc), result from several causes. For example, reduced Tc-99m bound only weakly to chelated substances can, under certain conditions, form insoluble technetium dioxide (TcO$_2$). Also, stannous ions, which normally serve as the reducing agent in Tc-99m kits, may undergo hydrolysis to form insoluble stannous hydroxide colloid, which can bind reduced Tc-99m. Significant amounts of HR-Tc are undesirable for several reasons: (1) the yield of the desired ^{99m}Tc-chelate is reduced by HR-Tc competing with the chelate for the available, reduced Tc-99m, and (2) image quality can be seriously degraded by the uptake of these colloidal impurities in organs of the RE system (liver, spleen, and bone marrow).

Thus, in the reduced Tc-99m agents, Tc-99m may be present in three distinct chemical forms:

1. "Free" (unbound) ^{99m}Tc-pertechnetate
2. "Hydrolyzed" Tc-99m (including reduced Tc-99m hydrolysis products *and* reduced Tc-99m bound to hydrolyzed Sn^{+2})
3. Bound Tc-99m chelate

Free, unbound pertechnetate and hydro-

---

*Labeling efficiency is the fraction of the radionuclide incorporated into the desired radiolabeled complex.

lyzed forms of Tc-99m in reduced Tc-99m radiopharmaceuticals are collectively known as radiochemical impurities. Optimally, their presence should be limited to trace quantities.

Fortunately, in most preparations the major fraction of Tc-99m radioactivity is in the desired, bound form; however, the accurate quantification of radiochemical impurities (by radiochromatographic analysis techniques) may occasionally be necessary. Analysis of radiochemical purity using radiochromatography is a quality control procedure discussed in Chapter 9.

8.4   RADIOISOTOPES OF IODINE

Radioisotopes of iodine are often used for radiolabeling many compounds that cannot be tagged with Tc-99m (Table 8–4). Among the 24 radioisotopes of iodine, only three (I-123, I-125, and I-131) have properties suitable for use in medicine (Table 8–5).

Generally, I-125 is limited (because of its relatively low-energy gamma emissions) to in vitro assay techniques such as radioimmunoassay procedures. I-131 (principal gamma emission 364 KeV) is useful for radiolabeling certain types of compounds (its 8.1-day physical half-life makes it suitable for radiolabeling compounds with slow uptake in target tissues). However, because I-131 is a beta-emitting radionuclide, usually only 1.0 mCi or less can be safely administered for diagnostic procedures.

I-123, because of its electron capture decay mode and principal photon emission of 159 KeV, is the most appealing of the iodine radioisotopes. Because it is an accelerator-produced radionuclide, however, it is relatively expensive. Also, its short physical half-life (13.3 hr) necessitates daily air delivery and limits usefulness for radiolabeling compounds that have lengthy target uptake or prolonged clearance from blood and background tissues.

Methods of Radioiodination

The process of labeling with radioiodine is known as radioiodination and is largely governed by the oxidation state of iodine (the I_2 state is necessary). For this reason the common property of all radioiodination methods involves the use of potent oxidizing substances, which, unfortunately, may damage the compound during labeling. This is of particular concern when radioiodinating certain materials, such as proteins, that require high specific activities and correspondingly severe oxidizing conditions for high-yield radioiodination. For radioiodination the pH may vary from 6 to 9, though radioiodination of proteins requires an alkaline pH.

In radioiodination, iodine binds firmly to aromatic compounds, with the primary binding site on proteins occurring at the tyrosyl group; the next important binding site is the imidazole ring of histidine.

Enzymatic Method. One of the most useful methods for protein radioiodination is an enzymatic method whereby enzymes (such as lactoperoxidase) release small quantities of hydrogen peroxide that oxidize iodide to its reactive state. Denaturation of proteins is usually minimal since only low concentrations of hydrogen per-

Table 8–4.   Radiopharmaceuticals that utilize radioisotopes of iodine.

Agent	Target Organ(s)/Tissues
^{131}I, ^{123}I-rose bengal	Liver (hepatobiliary)
^{131}I, ^{123}I-sodium ortho-iodohippurate	Kidneys
^{131}I-iodocholesterol	Adrenal cortex
^{131}I, ^{125}I-fibrinogen	Deep venous thrombosis

Table 8–5.   Radioisotopes of iodine useful in medicine.

	Physical Half-Life	Decay Mode	Principal Gamma Energy and Abundance	Detection Efficiency for ¼-inch NaI(Tl) Crystal
I-123	13.3 hr	EC	159 KeV (83%)	75%
I-125	60 days	EC	27.5 KeV (140%) 35 KeV (7%)	≈100%
I-131	8.1 days	β^-, γ	364 KeV (82%)	23%

oxide are formed. The relatively mild conditions for labeling and the high yields (60 to 75%) make this method useful for radioiodinating proteins and other compounds susceptible to denaturation.

Chloramine-T Method. The chloramine-T (N-chloro-p-toluenesulfonamide) method oxidizes iodide under somewhat more severe conditions than does the enzymatic method. While the labeling usually produces a high specific activity product, the labeling conditions may, even with carefully controlled concentrations of chloramine-T, cause some degree of product damage.

Excitation Labeling. Radioiodination by the excitation (or recoil) method is limited to I-123 and occurs when Xe-123 decays to form I-123. In this decay process, I-123 is a chemically reactive species because of recoil energy and will form bonds with many types of molecules. In the presence of chlorine, for instance, I-123 formed by the decay of Xe-123 produces ^{123}ICl, a reagent well suited to protein radioiodination.

Iodine Monochloride Method. For many years this was the primary method of radioiodination. Radioiodine is first equilibrated with stable iodine, which is usually in dilute HCl. This mixture is then added directly to the compound of interest for labeling at optimum pH and temperature. Since "cold" iodine is used, direct labeling with the nonradioactive iodine can also occur, thus lowering the specific activity of the labeled compound.

Other Methods. Electrolysis is another method useful for radioiodination. Electrolysis releases reactive iodine under relatively mild conditions and is an excellent

means for labeling many amino acids and proteins. Another radioiodination method employs chlorine gas or hypochloride in solution to oxidize iodide to the reactive iodine. These approaches also produce high labeling yields.

Precautions During Radioiodination

Elemental iodine is not highly soluble in aqueous solution and under certain conditions will volatilize, becoming a source of environmental contamination. Inhaled airborne radioiodine taken up by the thyroid gland can pose serious health concerns for nuclear pharmacy personnel. Atmospheric exhaust hoods should be used for liquid radioiodine storage or handling open containers of these materials.

8.5 METALLIC RADIONUCLIDES (THE TRANSITION METALS)

Of the remaining radioactive elements that can be used for radiolabeling, the radioisotopes of metallic elements are perhaps the most useful. Methods of radiolabeling and applications of several nonmetallic radionuclides, including radioisotopes of carbon, oxygen, and nitrogen, are discussed later in this chapter.

Characteristically, transition metals exist in multiple oxidation states, one or more of which are stable in water. The ability of metallic ions to form radiopharmaceutical complexes involves the unfilled outer electron shells, which enable the ions to either donate or receive electrons. For some radioactive metals a variety of radiopharmaceutical complexes have been developed, while for others only the simplest chemical forms (such as the salts) may be useful clinically. Since the biological distribution of the salt-type radiopharmaceuticals (such as Tl-201 thallous chloride and Ga-67 gallium citrate) is usually determined by their elemental properties, these agents are more appropriately discussed under their respective clinical applications.

Indium as a Radiolabel

Indium is a metallic element belonging to group III of the periodic chart (other members include aluminum, gallium, and thallium). In aqueous media, indium can be complexed with a wide variety of chelating agents that are useful in studying bone marrow and cerebrospinal fluid kinetics, and in blood pool imaging. Indium-labeled blood components—platelets and white blood cells—can be used to study physiologic functions such as blood clot formation and chemotactic response to bacterial infection. Among the radioisotopes of indium, two are useful in medicine (Table 8–6).

In-113m is a generator product obtained from the decay of parent Sn-113. Because of the long physical half-life of Sn-113 (115 days), a single generator may be useful for several months. The daughter, In-113m, with its physical half-life of 100 minutes and principal photon energy of 393 KeV, produces satisfactory images with the scintillation camera. In-113m was introduced for medical use as early as 1966 but has received only minimal attention because of the nearly ideal nuclear properties of gen-

erator-produced Tc-99m, which was developed shortly afterwards.

In-111 is a cyclotron product that is useful for the preparation of several radiopharmaceuticals. It decays by desirable electron capture, has highly abundant 173 and 247 KeV principal photons, which makes it well suited for use with the scintillation camera, and has a 2.8-day physical half-life, which makes it particularly desirable for studies requiring imaging as long as 2 to 3 days after injection. Although indium is an extremely toxic element, both In-111 and In-113m are carrier-free and may be safely administered (imaging doses usually contain less than $10^{-9}M$ elemental indium). In-111 radiopharmaceuticals presently include ^{111}In-DTPA, which is employed for the study of cerebrospinal fluid kinetics, and In-111 oxine, an agent used for labeling blood cell components, particularly leukocytes and platelets.

Radiolabeling Blood Cell Components with In-111

In serum, ionic indium, like iron, is rapidly affixed to circulating transferrin. When it is complexed to lipophilic chelates such as oxine (8-hydroxyquinoline), however, radioindium is directed away from hydrophilic sites such as transferrin to more lipophilic cellular components. When leukocytes, platelets, or lymphocytes are selectively isolated from whole blood and incubated with In-111 oxine under proper conditions, the radiopharmaceutical diffuses through the cell membrane, whereupon In-111 dissociates from oxine and forms tight bonds with intracellular cyto-

Table 8–6. Radioisotopes of indium useful in nuclear medicine.

	Physical Half-Life	Decay Mode	Principal Photons	
			Energy (KeV)	Abundance
In-111	2.8 days	EC	173	89%
			247	94%
In-113m*	1.7 hr	IT	393	64%

*Product of ^{113}Sn = ^{113m}In generator.

plasmic components. Nonradioactive oxine passes back outside the cell.

The selective isolation and labeling of blood cells with In-111 permits the accomplishment of a wide range of imaging procedures. For example, In-111–labeled platelets are useful for the detection of clots and vascular thrombi, while In-111–labeled leukocytes are widely used for the detection of abscesses. A brief description for the procedure for In-111 labeling of autologous leukocytes is shown in Figure 8–1.

8.6   CHROMIUM AS A RADIOLABEL

The transition metal chromium is often used in nuclear medicine for radiolabeling red blood cells (see Chapter 13) and pro-

teins such as human serum albumin. Cr-51 (Table 8–7) is the radioisotope of chromium employed for these procedures.

For in vitro labeling of red blood cells, 50 to 100 μCi of ^{51}Cr-sodium chromate ($Na_2{}^{51}CrO_4$) are mixed with whole blood and ACD solution (ACD stands for *Acid Citrate Dextrose*, a solution composed of citric acid, sodium citrate, and dextrose in water). The mixture is incubated in a water bath at 37° C for 20 minutes and shaken occasionally. Because only Cr(VI) binds red blood cells, any reduction in the chromium oxidation state from the active Cr(VI) state to the nonreactive Cr(III) state will halt the red cell labeling process. After incubation, the mixture is cooled at room temperature for 10 minutes, and 100 mg of ascorbic acid

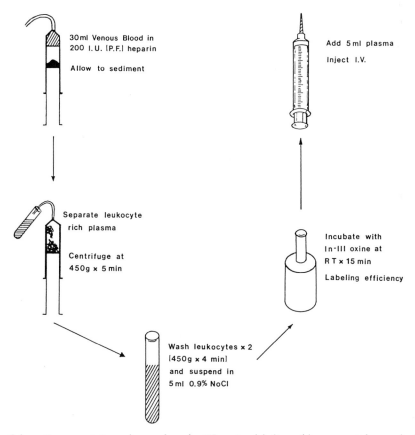

Fig. 8–1.   Schematic presentation of procedure for ^{111}In-oxine labeling of human autologous leukocytes for abscess localization. (From Thakur, ML, and Gottschalk, A: Experiences with Indium-111-oxine. *In* Indium-111 Labeled Neutrophils, Platelets, and Lymphocytes. Edited by ML Thakur, A Gottschalk. New York, Trivirum Publishing Co., 1980, p. 43, with permission.)

Table 8–7. Nuclear properties of Cr-51

	Physical Half-Life	Decay Mode	Principal Photons	
			Energy (KeV)	Abundance
Cr-51	27.8 days	EC	323	9%

are added to halt the reaction. The cells are washed (to remove unlabeled Cr-51) and resuspended in saline for injection. Generally, the red blood cell labeling yields are between 80 and 90%.

8.7 ORGANIC SYNTHESIS INVOLVING ACCELERATOR-PRODUCED RADIOISOTOPES OF CARBON, NITROGEN, AND OXYGEN

The basic concept of organic synthesis involves the introduction of a radioactive atom into a compound with known biological behavior. Usually, the preparation of these compounds involves substitution-type reactions in which radioisotopes of normally occurring elements (or their analogues) are placed into compounds. Because of the short physical half-life of C-11, N-13, and O-15—20, 10, and 2 minutes, respectively—the synthetic reactions necessary for the incorporation of the radionuclides must be rapid. Cyclotrons and the facilities for the chemical processing of these radionuclides must be in close proximity to the clinical sites.

The incorporation of radionuclides into some compounds can also be made by biological synthesis, or *biosynthesis*, whereby a living organism is grown in a culture medium that contains a radionuclide. Under carefully controlled conditions, the radionuclide is incorporated by normal metabolic processes into metabolites that can be chemically separated and are clinically useful. For example, cyanocobalamin (vitamin B_{12}) can be labeled with either Co-57 or Co-60 when these radionuclides are added to a culture medium in which *Streptomyces griseus* is grown. ^{75}Se-selenomethionine, a radiopharmaceutical employed for pancreas and thymus gland imaging, is also prepared by biosynthesis.

REFERENCES

1. DeKieviet, W: Technetium radiopharmaceuticals: chemical characterization and tissue distribution of Tc-glucoheptonate using Tc-99m and carrier Tc-99. J Nucl Med 22:703–709, 1981.
2. Eckelman, WC, Coursey, BM (eds).: Technetium-99m. Int J Appl Rad Isot 33:843–852, 1982.
3. Eckelman, WC, Levenson, SM: Radiopharmaceutical chemistry of technetium and iodine. *In* Textbook of Nuclear Medicine: Basic Science. Edited by AFG Rocha, HC Harbert. Philadelphia, Lea & Febiger, 1978, p. 192.
4. Howard, BY: Safe handling of radioiodinated solutions. J Nucl Med Tech 4:28–30, 1976.
5. Jones, AG, Davison, A: The relevance of basic technetium chemistry to nuclear medicine. J Nucl Med 23:1041–1043, 1982.
6. Mathias, CJ, Welch, MJ: Radiolabeling of platelets. Semin Nucl Med 14:118–127, 1984.
7. Richards, P, Steigman, J: Chemistry of technetium as applied to radiopharmaceuticals. *In* Radiopharmaceuticals, Edited by G Subramanian et al. New York, The Society of Nuclear Medicine, 1975, pp. 23–35.
8. Steigman, J, Richards, P: Chemistry of technetium-99m. Semin Nucl Med 4:269–279, 1974.
9. Thakur, ML, Gottschalk, A: Experience with Indium-111-oxine. *In* Indium-111 Labeled Neutrophils, Platelets, and Lymphocytes. Edited by ML Thakur, A Gottschalk. New York, Trivirum Publishing Co., 1980, pp. 41–50.
10. Thakur, ML, Seifert, CL, Madsen, MT, et al.: Neutrophil labeling: problems and pitfalls. Semin Nucl Med 14:107–117, April, 1984.

CHAPTER
9

Quality Control and Radiopharmaceuticals

In the broadest sense, the term "quality control" refers to the collective efforts made to assure the integrity of a particular substance, event, or situation. In nuclear medicine, quality control assurances for *radiopharmaceuticals* are intended to establish their desired biological and radiopharmaceutical character, while quality control procedures for *radiation detection instrumentation* assure the proper calibration of equipment, including accuracy of assay and imaging performance.

9.1 RADIOPHARMACEUTICAL QUALITY CONTROL

For radiopharmaceuticals, Briner has defined quality control as a "series of tests, analyses, and observations which establish beyond reasonable doubt the identity, quality, and quantity of a product's ingredients and which will demonstrate that the technology employed in its formulation will yield a dosage form of highest safety, purity, and efficacy." Assurances of radiopharmaceutical quality control, which involve tests of *biological purity* and *radiopharmaceutical character*, will be discussed first.

9.2 TESTS OF BIOLOGICAL PURITY FOR RADIOPHARMACEUTICALS

The vast majority of radiopharmaceuticals are administered intravenously. Therefore, radiopharmaceuticals, like most traditional pharmaceuticals, must be tested for *sterility* and *apyrogenicity* according to

Food and Drug Administration (FDA) guidelines. These tests are usually performed by the manufacturer, though nuclear pharmacy personnel may occasionally be required to test these two parameters on special products formulated in the nuclear pharmacy.

9.3 STERILITY

The term "sterility" indicates the absence of any viable microorganism.

Methods of Sterilization. The most familiar method of sterilization is steam "autoclaving." In this process, steam heating at 121° C is applied at 18 lb per square inch for 15 to 20 minutes. Materials such as glassware, utensils, and some solutions that can withstand these conditions are routinely sterilized by steam autoclaving, but materials that are damaged by high temperatures require other means of sterilization. For heat-labile solutions, the preferred method for sterilization is filtration through a membrane filter, which removes (by sieving action) microorganisms larger than the diameter of the filter pore. Membrane filters, composed of cellulose esters, are most commonly employed for this purpose and are available in several pore sizes. The preferred filter pore size for sterilization of solutions is 0.22 μ. Sterilization by membrane filtration is simple to perform, relatively inexpensive, and practical with a variety of solutions and substances.

Other sterilization methods include irradiation with high doses of gamma rays or exposure to gaseous ethylene oxide. Both of these methods can be used satisfactorily with heat-sensitive nonliquids such as plastic syringes and IV tubing.

Testing for Sterility. According to the United States Pharmacopeia XXI, sterility tests are performed by innoculating growth media, storing the innoculated media under conditions suitable for the growth of the contaminating microorganisms, and periodically checking the media for microbial growth. Fluid thioglycollate media (FTM) incubated at 30 to 35° C is used to check for facultative aerobic and anaerobic bacteria, while soybean casein digest media is used to test for fungi, molds, and aerobic and facultative anaerobic bacteria. Depending upon the method of final product packaging and preparation, the innoculated media is observed over 3 to 14 days, and the presence of any microorganisms is considered a positive result. Unfortunately, this method is slow and requires culture equipment and experienced personnel for proper operation.

Another method for sterility determinations involves the innoculation of culture media containing ^{14}C-glucose, which, in the presence of fermenting bacteria, results in the production of radiolabeled $^{14}CO_2$ detectable by an automated radiometric assay system. Using this method, sterility can be determined within 24 hours. Sterility testing using radiometric assay has some disadvantages: it is not yet officially recognized as a replacement for standard culture media techniques, and false negative results may occur because some bacteria do not emit CO_2.

9.4 PYROGENICITY

Pyrogens are heat-stable, filterable, soluble substances that produce symptoms of fever, chills, joint pain, headaches, and other complaints following IV injection. Pyrogenic reactions develop in patients between 30 minutes and 2 hours following administration of materials contaminated by pyrogens; they are rarely fatal and usually subside within a day. The usual pyrogens are products of gram-negative bacterial cell walls, so-called endotoxin, although pyrogenic reactions can also be caused by chemicals that have pyrogenic properties. The most common source of endotoxin is the surface of glassware used in product preparation or manufacture.

Sterility does not guarantee apyrogenicity and sterilization does not destroy pyrogens. Application of very high dry heat (250° F) for not less than 30 minutes is the desired method for rendering materials pyrogen free.

Testing for Apyrogenicity. Until recently the USP Pyrogen Test was the specified method for determining apyrogenicity. Briefly, this test required the injection of a test sample into the ear vein of three mature healthy rabbits with rectal temperatures measured at 1, 2, and 3 hours after injection. If no individual rabbit showed a temperature increase of 0.6° C or more, and if the sum of the temperature increases of all three animals did not exceed 1.4° C, the test sample was considered apyrogenic. If not, the test had to be repeated in five more rabbits and the results for all eight rabbits pooled. If not more than three of the total eight animals had individual temperature increases of 0.6° C or more and the sum of all eight temperature increases did not exceed 3.7° C, the material was accepted by USP standards as apyrogenic.

Rabbits are used for pyrogen testing because of their extreme sensitivity to pyrogenic substances. Because they are subject to temperature elevations solely from fright or excitation, however, they must be challenged frequently with known pyrogens to verify their sensitivity.

Recently, USP XXI has specified a new test, the Limulus Amebocyte Lysate (LAL) test, as a replacement for the older method of pyrogen testing. The principle of the LAL pyrogen test was established several years ago when it was shown that solutions of the amebocytes from the blood of the horseshoe crab, *Limulus polyphemus*, form an opaque gel when incubated with pyrogens. In medicine, the value of the LAL pyrogen test went largely unnoticed until recently, when the sensitivity of the LAL test for pyrogens was shown in a clinically related situation. During the mid-1960s, radioiodinated (I-131) human serum albumin (RISA) given to patients who subsequently developed aseptic meningitis yielded positive test results by LAL analysis yet had originally tested negative for pyrogens with the rabbit test method. These results, which indicated the much greater sensitivity of the LAL test for pyrogens, stimulated additional testing and refinement of the procedure. Subsequently, the LAL test for pyrogens has been shown preferable to the rabbit test method for the testing of radiopharmaceuticals because:

1. it can be performed in-house with minimal equipment and personnel
2. test volumes may be as small as 0.1 ml
3. the LAL test is completed within an hour
4. both positive and negative controls can be performed with each test
5. it is relatively inexpensive and the test materials may be stored until needed. Also, the greater sensitivity of the LAL test allows dilution of the test sample up to 1:50 (except for certain materials to be administered intrathecally).

The LAL test procedure is briefly outlined in Table 9–1.

9.5 TESTS OF RADIOPHARMACEUTICAL CHARACTER

In addition to the quality control considerations for sterility and apyrogenicity, other radiopharmaceutical quality control tests include tests for radionuclidic purity, radiochemical purity, and chemical purity.

Radionuclide Purity

Radionuclidic purity is defined as the proportion of total radioactivity present as the stated radionuclide. A radionuclidic impurity, therefore, is a radionuclide other than the one that is desired. The undesirable radionuclide(s) may be either a radioisotope of the desired radionuclide (same number of protons, different atomic mass) or a radioactive form of another element. Examples of radionuclidic impurities include unbound (free) radioiodides (such as I-131 and I-124) that occur in the preparation of I-123, and Mo-99 that is present in ^{99m}Tc-sodium pertechnetate.

Testing for Radionuclide Purity. For most radionuclides, radionuclidic purity can be determined by measuring either physical half-lives or characteristic gamma ray emissions. Evaluation of gamma ray emissions via pulse-height spectra (Fig. 9–1) permits identification of gamma ray energies and verification of purity according to guidelines provided by regulatory agencies. The radiopharmaceutical manufacturer usually has the responsibility of assuring radionuclidic purity.

Table 9–1.   Outline of test procedure and results for controls and test samples of LAL test for pyrogens.

LAL TUBE*	TEST SAMPLE OR CONTROL	RESULTS OR COMMENTS
#1	Negative Control (pyrogen-free saline)	Should be negative
#2	Positive Control (endotoxin[t])	Should be positive
#3	Positive Internal Control (test sample tainted with endotoxin[t])	Should be positive—useful in demonstrating integrity of LAL test with test sample
#4	Test Sample	May be positive or negative

Test Conditions: All samples should be incubated at 37° C for 1 hour following addition of test samples/controls to LAL tubes. LAL reactivity is optimum at neutral pH values.

*Each LAL tube contains 0.1 ml amebocyte lysate; each tube should be duplicated.
[t]Usually *E. coli*

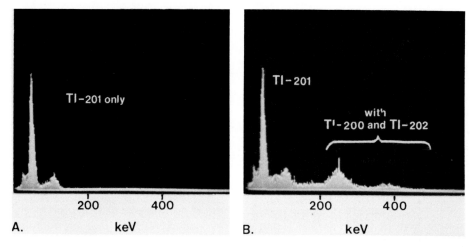

Fig. 9–1. Comparison of pulse-height spectra for radioisotopically pure Tl-201 (A) and Tl-201 containing radionuclidic contaminants (B).

Sources of radionuclidic impurities may include poor separation techniques (failure to remove during processing all but the desired radioactive product). Often, such impurities may originate from contaminants in the target that are activated during target bombardment.

In the production of some radionuclides, radionuclidic impurities are generated as a consequence of the production reaction. Usually, these radionuclidic impurities are of no consequence since they often have relatively short physical half-lives (compared to the half-life of the desired radionuclide). However, during production of some radionuclides certain characteristic radionuclidic impurities can be produced that are longer-lived than the principal radionuclide. In these situations, the relative fraction of radioactivity represented by the longer-lived radionuclide impurity actually increases with time, since the shorter-lived principal radionuclide is decaying more rapidly. An example is I-123 contaminated with longer-lived radioisotopes of iodine (Fig. 9–2).

Assay for Mo-99 Content in ⁹⁹Mo-⁹⁹ᵐTc Generator Eluate. In order to assure that Mo-99 levels in generator eluate do not exceed maximum allowable levels (Table 9–2), each ⁹⁹Mo-⁹⁹ᵐTc generator eluate must

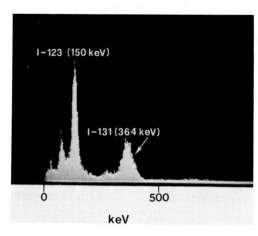

Fig. 9–2. Pulse-height spectra of a sample of I-123 containing I-131.

be assayed for Mo-99 content. Mo-99 assay can be accomplished by one of two methods.

1. The *lead shield method*, the most commonly used method, is performed by placing the generator eluate in a specially constructed lead container (Fig.

Table 9–2. Maximum allowable activities of Mo-99 in Tc-99m generator eluate (USP XXI).

—No more than 0.15 μCi Mo-99 per each Mo-99 at time of patient administration

*Some regulatory agencies have maintained the Mo-99 limits at 1.0 μCi Mo-99 per each mCi Tc-99m, or no more than 5 μCi Mo-99 per patient dose.

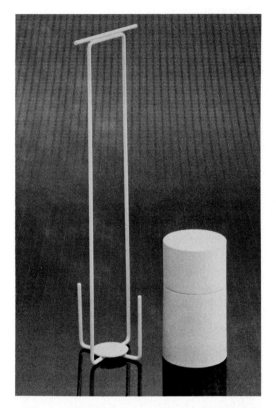

Fig. 9–3. Lead shield used for assaying Mo-99 activity in ⁹⁹Mo-⁹⁹ᵐTc generator eluate. Shield is ¼-inch thick lead. The shield can be placed directly in a radionuclide dose calibrator by using the cradle (shown on the left).

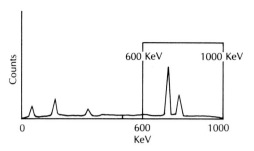

Fig. 9–4. Pulse-height analysis (PHA) of Mo-99. Principal photons of Mo-99 (740 and 780 KeV) can be adequately quantified by integrating instrument to "count" photons emitted in the 600 to 1000 KeV range.

9–3) for Mo-99 assay. These containers, which have lead walls approximately ¼ inch thick, effectively absorb the lower-energy Tc-99m emissions (140 KeV) yet permit the passage of approximately one half of the more energetic Mo-99 photons (740 and 780 KeV). With the shielded generator eluate placed in a radionuclide dose calibrator, the Mo-99 content can be assayed directly. With many of the older radionuclide dose calibrators, however, it is necessary to multiply the Mo-99 assay by a conversion factor (usually two), since only one half the Mo-99 activity is measured. Newer dose calibrators automatically correct for this attenuation.

2. The *alternative Mo-99 assay method* compares the unknown Mo-99 activity to that of a reference standard (usually Cs-137). The radiation detection instrument is a well-type detector system connected to a gamma ray spectrometer. With the pulse-height analyzer of the instrument set to accept only those counts within the 600 to 1000 KeV range (Fig. 9–4), the number of photons occurring in this range is determined for the generator eluate. The generator vial is removed from the lead shield, and a Cs-137 standard source (principal photon energy 662 KeV) is counted in this same 600 to 1000 KeV range and under identical conditions. Since in this energy range the numbers of photons emitted by equal activities of Cs-137 and Mo-99 differ by a factor of approximately 4.25 (Fig. 9–5), it is possible to establish ratios of counts per minute/μCi and calculate Mo-99 activity.

Other Radionuclide Contaminants. Occasionally, generators prepared from fission-product Mo-99 may contain small amounts of fission by-products that may be eluted from the generator column. These radionuclidic impurities include I-131, Zr-99, Te-132, Ru-103, Sb-124, Cs-134, and Rb-86. Limits have been set for these contaminants (USP XXI)—no more

	Mo-99	Cs-137
Principal Photons:	740 & 780 KeV	662 KeV
Abundance:	12% + 8% = 20%	85%

Relative Value (600–1000 KeV range):	$\dfrac{\text{Cs-137 principal photons}}{\text{Mo-99 principal photons}} = \dfrac{85\%}{20\%} = \boxed{4.25}$

Fig. 9–5. Comparison of relative abundance of principal photons of Mo-99 and Cs-137 (between 600 and 1000 KeV). Relative value shown valid for comparison of equal activities of Mo-99 and Cs-137.

than 0.5 μCi for each mCi Tc-99m and no more than 2.5 μCi per administered dose.

Radiochemical Purity

Radiochemical purity is defined as the fraction of total radioactivity present in the desired chemical form. For example, in Tc-99m radiopharmaceuticals the presence of Tc-99m in any other chemical form constitutes a radiochemical impurity.

In the case of most Tc-99m radiopharmaceuticals two principal radiochemical impurities can exist— free (unbound) ^{99m}Tc-pertechnetate, and hydrolyzed, reduced Tc-99m (which occurs only in the reduced Tc[IV] radiopharmaceuticals).

Radiochemical impurities are not limited to Tc-99m radiopharmaceuticals; for example, free I-131 occurring in ^{131}I-labeled agents would also be a radiochemical impurity. Radiochemical impurities are undesirable for two reasons. First, the scintigraphic appearance of radiochemical impurities in blood and nontarget organs can seriously affect image quality by lowering target/nontarget ratios (Fig. 9–6). Second, radiochemical impurities increase patient radiation exposure by their concentration in certain organs and tissues.

Radiochromatographic Analysis for Determining Radiochemical Purity. Radiochemical purity is best determined using *radiochromatographic analysis* techniques (often called *thin layer chromatography*, or TLC), that employ solvent separation techniques for the fractionation of radiochemical components. In this method, a small drop of the radiopharmaceutical is "spot-

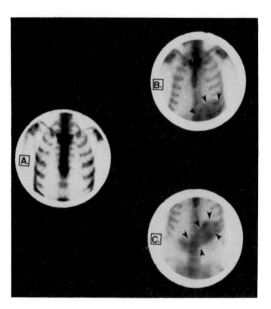

Fig. 9–6. Scintiphotos of patients injected with ^{99m}Tc-medronate, a bone-seeking radiopharmaceutical. Scintiphoto A shows a high quality skeletal image of an anterior chest. Scintiphoto B shows a much poorer quality image of an anterior chest. Noted in the left lower quadrant *(arrows)* is radiopharmaceutical uptake suggestive of stomach. In Scintiphoto C, this area of uptake is confirmed to be stomach. Uptake of the radiopharmaceutical in the stomach during bone imaging is primarily caused by the presence of high levels of free (unbound) pertechnetate in the bone imaging radiopharmaceutical.

ted" onto a support medium (either a strip of paper or a fiberglass/silica gel matrix) at a point near one end. The strip is placed ("spotted" end first) in a container holding a small amount of a desired solvent. As the solvent migrates by capillary forces along the media strip, soluble components "move" with the solvent while insoluble components remain at the point of application (i.e., the *origin*). Usually, 3 to 5 min-

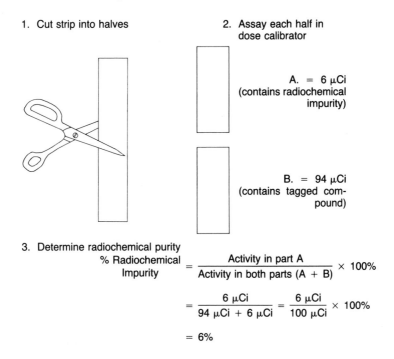

1. Cut strip into halves

2. Assay each half in dose calibrator

A. = 6 μCi
(contains radiochemical impurity)

B. = 94 μCi
(contains tagged compound)

3. Determine radiochemical purity

$$\frac{\text{\% Radiochemical}}{\text{Impurity}} = \frac{\text{Activity in part A}}{\text{Activity in both parts (A + B)}} \times 100\%$$

$$= \frac{6\ \mu Ci}{94\ \mu Ci + 6\ \mu Ci} = \frac{6\ \mu Ci}{100\ \mu Ci} \times 100\%$$

$$= 6\%$$

Fig. 9–7. "Cut and assay" method for quantifying radiochemical impurity using radiochromatography.

utes are required for the solvent to reach the top of the media strip (i.e., the *solvent front*), depending upon the strip length and type of solvent used.

When the solvent reaches the solvent front, the strip is removed and allowed to dry. Later, the strip is cut in half and each half is assayed for the amount of radioactivity (Fig. 9–7). A radionuclide dose calibrator is usually adequate for this purpose. Alternatively, a radiochromatogram scanner (Fig. 9–8) can detect and measure the distribution of radioactivity along the intact radiochromatography strip (Fig. 9–9).

The specific solvent systems and support media necessary to separate various components depends on the radiopharmaceutical to be tested and the potential radiochemical impurities present. Solvent/media radiochromatography systems for selected Tc-99m radiopharmaceuticals are shown in Table 9–3.

Radiochromatographic analysis techniques provide a direct measurement of the amount of radiochemical impurity present;

the "tagging" efficiency may be determined by the following formula:

$$\frac{\text{Tagging}}{\text{Efficiency}} = 100\% - (\% \text{ radiochemical impurities})$$

In the case of selected Tc-99m radiopharmaceuticals, the tagging efficiency is determined indirectly, as follows:

$$\frac{\text{Tagging}}{\text{Efficiency}} = 100\% - (\% \text{ free } ^{99m}\text{TcO}_4^-$$
$$+ \% \text{ hydrolyzed, reduced } ^{99m}\text{Tc})$$

Factors Affecting Radiochemical Purity. Radiochemical purity depends on the ability of the radiolabeled complex to resist degradation. Factors that can be responsible for deterioration include change in pH, improper storage conditions (exposure to light or extreme temperatures), poor preparation technique, the passage of time, and the presence of oxidants or reducing agents. Optimum storage conditions and pH values for selected radiopharmaceuticals (according to USP XXI) are shown in Table 9–4. Minimum radiochemical purity requirements for selected radiopharmaceuticals are shown in Table 9–5.

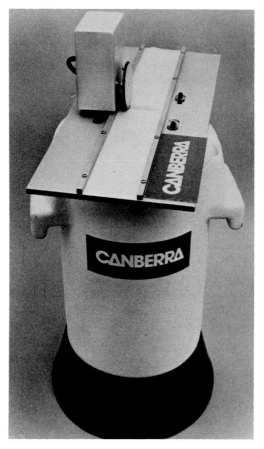

Fig. 9–8. Radiochromatogram scanner shown with a well-type detector. The unit drives the radiochromatogram strip over the detector at a constant speed that allows the radioactivity along the strip to be analyzed and plotted by a multichannel analyzer (not shown). (Courtesy of Canberra.)

Chemical Purity

Chemical impurities are nonradioactive substances that may affect either radiopharmaceutical biodistribution or product integrity. For example, aluminum ions from the generator column occasionally found in significant quantities in the Tc-99m eluate (alumina breakthrough) have been reported to cause the formation of undesirably large particles of ^{99m}Tc-sulfur colloid, which are taken up by the lungs instead of by the RE system. Additionally, alumina breakthrough has also been indi-

cated as responsible for altered biodistribution of other Tc-99m radiopharmaceuticals (Table 9–6). Aluminum ions in generator eluate can be identified using a colorimetric assay method (Fig. 9–10), which detects levels greater than 10 µg Al^{+3}/ml (the established limit for Al^{+3} ions in the generator eluate). With the present generator technology, alumina breakthrough occurs only rarely.

9.6 CALIBRATION OF RADIONUCLIDE DOSE CALIBRATOR

The radionuclide dose calibrator is used routinely in the clinical nuclear medicine laboratory to measure radiopharmaceutical doses prior to patient administration. Except for radiopharmaceuticals that contain either pure beta-emitting radionuclides or less than 10 µCi of 9 gamma-emitting radionuclide, all other radiopharmaceuticals must be assayed for the amount of radioactivity prior to patient administration. Additionally, these dosages must be within ± 10% of the radioactivity intended to be administered. To ensure proper dose measurement and functioning of the radionuclide dose calibrator, this instrument must be calibrated periodically according to NRC guidelines. There are four required tests of calibration for radionuclide dose calibrators (Table 9–7).

Test of Instrument Linearity

The linearity of the dose calibrator involves the ability of the instrument to correctly assay both large and small amounts of radioactivity. The test of instrument linearity is performed by assaying a source of Tc-99m equivalent to the maximum activity normally used, then assaying it again 6, 24, 30, and 48 hours later.

Using the 30-hour activity assay as the starting point, the decay-predicted values

A.

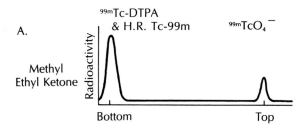

Methyl
Ethyl Ketone

B.

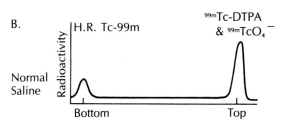

Normal
Saline

Fig. 9–9. Radiochromatography strips spotted with ^{99m}Tc-DTPA and developed with methyl ethyl ketone (Strip A) and normal saline (Strip B) and processed with a radiochromatogram scanner device. Specific radiochemical components are shown on each radiochromatographic strip following migration with the specified solvent system.

H.R. Tc-99m = hydrolyzed, reduced technetium (colloidal)

^{99m}TcO$_4^-$ = free, unbound pertechnetate

Table 9–3.   Radiochromatography techniques for selected Tc-99m radiopharmaceuticals.

| | | | rF Values* | | |
Radiopharmaceutical	Support Media	Solvent	Radio-pharmaceutical	Free ^{99m}TcO$_4$	HR^t ^{99m}Tc
^{99m}Tc-sulfur colloid	Gelman ITLC-SG	0.9% NaCl	0.0	0.9	N.A.
^{99m}Tc-macroaggregated albumin	Gelman ITLC-SG	0.9% NaCl	0.0	0.9	N.A.
^{99m}Tc-sodium pertechnetate	Whatman 31 ET	Acetone**	0.0	0.9	0.0
^{99m}Tc-pentetate (DTPA)	Whatman 31 ET	Methyl Ethyl Ketone	0.0	0.9	0.0
	Gelman ITLC-SG	0.9% NaCl	1.0	1.0	0.0
^{99m}Tc-pyrophosphate	Whatman 31 ET	Methyl Ethyl Ketone	0.0	1.0	0.0
	Gelman ITLC-SG	0.9% NaCl	1.0	1.0	0.0
^{99m}Tc-medronate (MDP)	Whatman 31 ET	Methyl Ethyl Ketone	0.0	0.9	0.0
	Gelman ITLC-SG	0.9% NaCl	1.0	1.0	0.0
^{99m}Tc-oxidronate (HMDP)	Whatman 31 ET	Acetone	0.0	0.9	0.0
	Gelman ITLC-SG	0.9% NaCl	1.0	1.0	0.0
^{99m}Tc-gluceptate	Whatman 31 ET	Acetone	0.0	0.9	0.0
	Gelman ITLC-SG	0.9% NaCl	1.0	1.0	0.0
^{99m}Tc-succimer (DMSA)	Gelman ITLC-SA	Acetone	0.0	1.0	0.0
^{99m}Tc-2,6-diisopropyl IDA	Gelman ITLC-SA	Saturated NaCl	0.0	1.0	0.0
(disofenin)	Gelman ITLC-SG	Distilled: H$_2$O (3:1)	1.0	1.0	0.0

*
rF Value = $\dfrac{\text{distance component travels from origin}}{\text{distance of solvent front from origin}}$

^{t}HR Tc-99m = hydrolyzed, reduced Tc-99m and includes all colloidal species of reduced Tc-99m
**Methyl ethyl ketone (MEK) may be used in place of acetone and vice versa

Table 9–4. Optimum storage conditions and pH values for selected radiopharmaceuticals (USP XXI).

Radiopharmaceutical	Storage Conditions	pH
[67]Ga-citrate injection	Single-dose or multidose containers	4.5–8.0
[99m]Tc-gluceptate	Single-dose or multidose containers 2°–8°C	4.0–8.0
[99m]Tc-macroaggregted albumin	Single-dose or multidose containers 2°–8°C	3.8–8.0
[99m]Tc-medronate (MDP)	Single-dose or multidose containers	4.0–7.8
[99m]Tc-oxidronate (HMDP)	Single-dose or multidose containers	2.5–7.0
[99m]Tc-penetate (DTPA)	Single-dose or multidose containers 2°–8°C	3.8–7.5
[99m]Tc-pyrophosphate	Single-dose or multidose containers 2°–8°C	4.0–7.5
[99m]Tc-sodium pertechnetate	Single-dose or multidose containers	4.5–7.5
[99m]Tc-succimer (DMSA)	Single-dose container 15°–30°C; protect from light	2.0–3.0
[99m]Tc-sulfur colloid	Single-dose or multidose containers	4.7–7.5
[123]I-sodium iodide solution	Single-dose or multidose containers	7.5–9.0
[131]I-sodium iodide solution	Single-dose or multidose containers	7.5–9.0
[131]I-sodium iodohippurate injection (OIHA)	Single-dose or multidose containers	7.0–8.5

Table 9–5. Minimum values of radiochemical purity for selected radiopharmaceuticals (from USP XXI). Values shown are minimum percentages of radioactivity present in desired radiochemical form.

85% minimum purity:
  ^{99m}Tc-succimer (DMSA)
90% minimum purity:
  ^{99m}Tc-pentetate (DTPA)
  ^{99m}Tc-sodium pertechnetate
  ^{99m}Tc-pyrophosphate
  ^{99m}Tc-macroaggregated albumin
92% minimum purity:
  ^{99m}Tc-sulfur colloid
97% minimum purity:
  ^{131}I-orthoiodohippuric acid (OIHA)

Assay Time (hr)		Correction Factors
0		31.63
6		15.85
24		1.99
30	..."STARTING" POINT...	1.00
48		0.126

EXAMPLE
If the net activity measured at 30 hr was 31.3 mCi, then the predicted activity at the other times would be equivalent to 31.3 mCi times the appropriate correction factor.

The assayed net activity for the sample at each time interval is plotted against the predicted activity (corrected for decay) on semilog paper (Fig. 9–11). If the dose calibrator is functioning properly, the assayed activities should be within ± 5% of the decay-predicted curve (using the 30-hr starting point). Differences greater than ± 5% indicate the need for instrument repair or adjustment.

Test for Geometric Variation. Changes

are calculated at 0-, 6-, 24-, and 48-hour time points using the following correction factors (alternatively, concentric lead shields of appropriate thickness can be used during assay to provide the desired values):

Table 9–6. Reported alterations of radiopharmaceutical biodistribution caused by aluminum ions.*

Agent	Reported Alteration
[99m]Tc-sulfur colloid	Lung uptake secondary to increase in particle size
[99m]Tc-phosphonates	Uptake in RE system
[99m]Tc-sodium pertechnetate	Failure of agent "to leave vascular space"

*For comprehensive listing of drug-induced alterations see Hladik, WB III, Nigg, KK, Rhodes, BA: Drug-induced changes in the biologic distribution of radiopharmaceuticals. Sem Nucl Med *12*(2):184–213, April 1982.

Table 9–7. Tests of calibration for radionuclide dose calibrators and the required frequency of testing.

Description	Testing Frequency
1. Test of instrument linearity	On installation, then quarterly
2. Test of geometric variation	On installation
3. Test of instrument accuracy	On installation
4. Test of instrument constancy	Daily

Procedure:
1. Place a 10 μl drop of eluate to be tested onto test paper strip.
2. Place similar size drop of standard Al^{+3} solution adjacent to eluate sample.
3. If intensity of center spot of sample is less than that for center of standard Al^{+3} solution, eluate contains less than 10 μg Al^{+3}/ml.

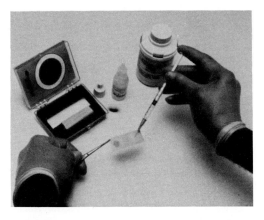

Fig. 9–10. Colorimetric assay method for the determination of Al^{+3} ions in ^{99}Mo-^{99m}Tc generator eluate.

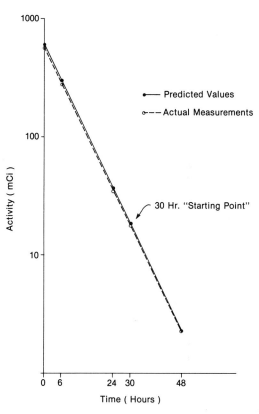

Fig. 9–11. Graphical display of results for a test of instrument linearity for a radionuclide dose calibrator. Actual measurements of radioactivity are plotted against predicted values using the assay values obtained at the 30-hour time as the "starting" point (all assay values in this example are within the desired ± 5% range of predicted assay values).

in sample volumes or geometric configuration of doses within the ionization chamber of the dose calibrator may affect the accuracy of measurements. The extent of these effects should be determined and, if variations are significant (greater than ± 2% of the "true" assay), appropriate correction factors may be necessary.

The test for geometric variation uses a 30-ml vial that contains 2 to 5 mCi of Tc-99m in a small volume (usually 1.0 ml or less). Net activity (minus background) of the vial is measured initially, then again after each increase in volume, using either normal saline or distilled water to 2, 4, 8, 10, 20, and 25 ml. A volume is then selected as "standard," and for each volume the ra-

tios of measured activity to the selected standard activity are calculated.

Test of Instrument Accuracy

Upon installation, the accuracy of the radionuclide dose calibrator is checked for several radionuclides (such as Cs-137 and

Co-57) using appropriate radionuclide sources whose activity was originally calibrated against a standard certified by the National Bureau of Standards (NBS). Measurements of the reference sources, usually taken as an average of three readings, should agree within ± 5% of the certified activity of the reference source. Variations greater than ± 5% indicate the need for instrument adjustment or repair.

Tests of Instrument Constancy

Daily checks with long-lived NBS reference sources, such as Cs-137, Co-57, Co-60, and Ra-226, are useful in evaluating the constancy of instrument measurement. A log should be maintained plotting daily assays against predicted decay activities (according to certified activities). Variations greater than ± 5% indicate the need for instrument adjustment or repair.

REFERENCES

1. Briner, WH: Quality control of radiopharmaceuticals. *In* Radioisotope in Pharmakokinetik und Klinischer Biochemie. Edited by W Keiderling, G Hoffman, HA Ladner, FK Stutgart. Schattauer Verlag 1970, pp. 37–46.
2. Anderson, DW, Raeside, DE, Ficken, VJ: Determination of impurity activities in fission-product generator eluate. J Nucl Med 15:889–891, 1974.
3. Billinghurst, MW, Palser, RF: Some factors affecting the calibration of radionuclide dose calibrators—I. ^{99m}Tc. Int J Nucl Med Biol 10:117–119, 1983.
4. Cooper, JF, Harbert, JC: Endotoxin as a cause of asceptic meningitis after radionuclide cisternography. J Nucl Med 16:809–813, 1975.
5. Cooper, JF: Pyrogen testing: Practical considerations. *In* Quality Assurance of Pharmaceuticals Manufactured in The Hospital. Edited by A Warbick-Cerone, LG Johnston. Dublin, Pergammon Press, 1985, p. 123–132.
6. Eckelman, WC: Radiochemical purity of new radiopharmaceuticals (editorial). J Nucl Med 17:865, 1976.
7. Eckelman, WC, Richards, P: Analytical pitfalls with ^{99m}Tc-labeled compounds. J Nucl Med 13:202–205, 1973.
8. Kowalsky, RJ, Johnston, RE, Chan, FH: Dose calibrator performances and quality control. J Nucl Med Tech 5:35–40, 1977.
9. Krohn, KA, Jansholt, AL: Radiochemical quality control of short-lived radiopharmaceuticals. Int J Appl Radiat Isot 28:213–227, 1977.
10. Rhodes, BA: Radiometric sterility testing. *In* Quality Control in Nuclear Medicine. Edited by BA Rhodes. St. Louis, CV Mosby Co., 1977, pp. 226–228.
11. Srivastava, SC, Meinken, G, Smith, TD, et al.: Problems associated with stannous ^{99m}Tc-radiopharmaceuticals. Int J Appl Radiat Isot 28:83–95, 1977.
12. Williams, CC, Kereiakes, JG, Grossman, LW: The accuracy of ^{99}Molybdenum assays in ^{99m}Technetium solutions. Radiology 138:445–448, 1981.
13. Zimmer, AM, Pavel, DG: Rapid miniaturized chromatographic quality-control procedures for Tc-99m radiopharmaceuticals. J Nucl Med 18:1230–1233, 1977.

Radiopharmaceuticals for Brain Imaging

10.1 BRAIN IMAGING

Nuclear medicine brain imaging (NMBI) is a screening procedure for the detection of cerebral pathology as reflected by alteration in regional blood-brain barrier permeability (static imaging) or by displacement and alterations in distribution of vascular perfusion (dynamic imaging).

Principle

Under normal circumstances the capillaries of the brain restrict exchange of many chemical substances from blood into the extravascular spaces surrounding the capillaries. This phenomenon of selective permeability is referred to as the blood-brain barrier (BBB). The BBB is permeable to a limited number of metabolic substrates, which are made up almost exclusively of the elements carbon, hydrogen, oxygen and nitrogen. Radiolabeled analogues of these substances would be useful in assessing cerebral physiology and pathology, but no suitable radioisotopes of these elements exist for general use in medicine. While the lipid nature of the BBB (Table 10–1) does permit passive permeability to a host of lipophilic substances (several of which can be labeled with gamma-emitting radionuclides), conventional brain imaging is performed with water-soluble radiopharmaceuticals. These agents do not penetrate the intact BBB into normal brain, crossing only the damaged BBB in pathologic processes, such as cerebral infarction, inflammation, and tumor,

Table 10–1. Influence of the blood-brain barrier (BBB) on permeability of various substances in blood.

  I. *BBB forms nonpermeable passive barrier*
     Macromolecules, charged-ions species, nonmetabolizable solutes.
 II. *BBB is freely passive to permit diffusion*
     Highly lipid soluble substances with octanol/H_2O partition coefficient greater than 0.03 (e.g., ethanol, xenon, amphetamines).
III. *BBB contains active carrier transport mechanisms*
     Active metabolic substrates (such as D-glucose, amino acids).

and they appear on scintillation images as focal areas of increased localization. This "uptake" (or concentration) of radiopharmaceutical in brain lesions is also influenced to a lesser extent by increased regional blood pools, increased extracellular fluid volume, and edema.

Indications

Although the NMBI study is useful in several clinical situations and is able to detect approximately 80 to 85% of intracranial

Table 10–2. Indications for brain imaging.

1. To screen patients for the presence of primary tumors, both benign and malignant.
2. To detect cerebral metastases.
3. To evaluate patients with cerebrovascular disease.
4. To detect intracranial injury due to trauma, such as subdural hematoma, intracerebral hemorrhage.
5. To localize intracranial abscesses.
6. To localize arteriovenous malformations.
7. To study patients with many varied intracranial diseases, such as meningitis, encephalitis.
8. To determine legally defined "brain-death."

neoplasms, its use has decreased since contrast-enhanced computed tomography (CT) has proven more sensitive and to provide somewhat better anatomic localization. For these reasons, CT is presently the initial diagnostic imaging study used when cerebral disease is suspected. It is likely, however, that in the near future magnetic resonance imaging (MRI) may supplant CT as the imaging procedure of choice for suspected cerebral disease.

The foregoing should not be taken to indicate, however, that the NMBI study has no diagnostic value. Brain imaging has several clinical applications (Table 10–2).

Radiopharmaceutical Data

In essence, NMBI studies can be performed with any radiopharmaceutical that has suitable physical properties and that is normally excluded by the intact blood-brain barrier. A number of radioactive substances have been used and several new agents are under evaluation for NMBI. Tc-99m radiopharmaceuticals, however, are almost universally employed for NMBI because they can be administered in the relatively large doses (with acceptable radiation exposure) needed to achieve the high count rates required for dynamic brain blood flow studies and to obtain high-quality static images in reasonably short periods of time. These Tc-99m radiopharmaceuticals share the property of producing higher concentrations in the brain tumor compared to normal brain tissue (so-called tumor/brain ratio) at some time after administration.

Tc-99m Pertechnetate. For many years, ^{99m}Tc-sodium pertechnetate (Na^{99m}TcO$_4$) was the agent of choice for NMBI. It is a relatively inexpensive generator product obtained directly from the decay of Mo-99. A disadvantage of ^{99m}Tc-sodium pertechnetate is its relatively slow blood clearance rate, which necessitates a delay of several hours after injection before static brain images with adequate tumor/brain ratios can be obtained.

Tc-99m DTPA and Tc-99m Gluceptate. The blood clearance of these agents is more rapid than for ^{99m}Tc-sodium pertechnetate, allowing high tumor/blood and tumor/normal brain ratios to be achieved earlier after injection (1 hour as opposed to the 3 to 4 hours for pertechnetate). Some clinical evidence indicates that the convenience of earlier imaging with these agents may be coupled with a slightly higher tumor detection rate, particularly for ^{99m}Tc-gluceptate (compared to Tc-99m pertechnetate). For these reasons, ^{99m}Tc-gluceptate appears to be the current agent of choice for NMBI studies. Neither ^{99m}Tc-DTPA nor ^{99m}Tc-gluceptate are accumulated by the choroid plexus, salivary glands, or thyroid, and their distribution is not altered by the presence of tin (such as occurs with prior bone imaging with certain Tc-99m radiopharmaceuticals that contain high levels of tin ions; the mechanism of interference is discussed in Chapter 15).

The biodistribution characteristics of Tc-99m sodium pertechnetate, Tc-99m DTPA, and Tc-99m gluceptate are shown in Table 10–3.

Iodinated (I-123) Amphetamines. Recently, there has been interest in developing brain imaging agents that provide

Table 10–3. Biodistribution characteristics of Tc-99m radiopharmaceuticals.

Na ^{99m}TcO$_4$ (^{99m}Tc-sodium pertechnetate)
  Does not cross intact BBB.
  Loosely bound to serum proteins ($\cong$80%).
  Nonprotein-bound fraction is filtered (approximately 80% reabsorbed).
  Accumulates in salivary glands, stomach, thyroid gland, and choroid plexus.*
  Presence of Sn^{+2} ions in blood results in RBC binding by Tc-99m.

^{99m}Tc-pentetate (DTPA) and ^{99m}Tc-gluceptate
  Does not cross intact BBB.
  Rapid blood clearance.
  Not accumulated by choroid plexus, salivary glands, thyroid, or stomach.
  Renal excretion mode makes these agents also useful for renal imaging.

*Can be blocked by PO administration of 250 mg of potassium perchlorate 1 hr prior to imaging.

diagnostic information on physiological parameters, such as brain blood flow. Iodinated amphetamines (such as ^{123}I-N-iso-propyl-p-iodoamphetamine) are highly lipophilic compounds that are freely permeable to the brain and have a high extraction rate. In the brain, they are thought to localize intracellularly by binding amine receptor sites. This hypothesis is supported by the demonstration that nonradiolabeled isopropyl-p-iodoamphetamine inhibits the uptake of other amine substrates. Clinical investigation of this agent is under way.

F-18, C-11, labeled Deoxy-D-glucose (DDG). Either F-18 or C-11 can be used to radiolabel the glucose analogue, deoxy-D-glucose (DDG), to form a short-lived positron-emitting radiopharmaceutical that is useful for brain imaging with positron emission tomography (PET) units. The radiolabeled analogue undergoes transport from blood to the brain by the same carrier system and at similar rates as glucose. Once inside brain cells, DDG undergoes phosphorylation by the enzyme hexokinase; however, unlike glucose, DDG is unable to undergo the subsequent enzymatic steps of glycolysis and becomes metabolically trapped inside brain cells. PET images of radiolabeled DDG yield apparent data on glucose utilization and, hence, brain metabolic activity.

Method

It is common to perform the NMBI with the Tc-99m radiopharmaceuticals in two parts—the "flow" (or dynamic) study and the "static" imaging. In the "flow" part of the NMBI, the radiopharmaceutical is injected intravenously (rapidly as a bolus), usually in a small volume (less than 1 cc), and the scintillation camera records the flow of the radiopharmaceutical in blood through the vessels of the neck and brain (Fig. 10–1). Rapid sequential scintillation camera images are obtained at 1- to 2-second intervals using the projection most

likely to show the suspected clinical problem. Routine studies in adults are most often performed in the anterior position, while in children the posterior position may be preferred. Adults usually receive 15 to 25 mCi of the Tc-99m radiopharmaceutical.

Most studies suggest that the optimum time for delayed imaging with ^{99m}Tc-pertechnetate is 3 to 4 hours after injection; 1 to 1½ hours is appropriate for ^{99m}Tc-DTPA and ^{99m}Tc-glucepate (Figs. 10–2 and 10–3). Immediate static studies are useful in demonstrating highly vascular lesions such as arteriovenous malformations, which might not be seen on delayed imaging.

Multiple views (usually at least four) are routine for static NMBI studies.

Special Considerations/Patient Preparation

Uptake of Tc-99m pertechnetate by the choroid plexus, which happens in about 25% of patients, can mimic or obscure a brain lesion in that area of the brain; potassium perchlorate, however, competitively inhibits accumulation of the pertechnetate ion in the choroid plexus, as well as in the salivary glands and thyroid. A single, oral dose of 250 mg of potassium perchlorate given prior to imaging will prevent (block) choroid plexus uptake of Tc-99m pertechnetate. This form of patient preparation is necessary only for Tc-99m pertechnetate and not for the other Tc-99m radiopharmaceuticals.

10.2   CEREBROSPINAL FLUID (CSF) IMAGING

Nuclear medicine cerebrospinal fluid (CSF) imaging (or radionuclide cisternography) is a diagnostic procedure entailing sequential imaging of radiopharmaceutical distribution in the spinal and cranial CSF spaces following injection of the agent into the subarachnoid space. The procedure is based on the assumption that the move-

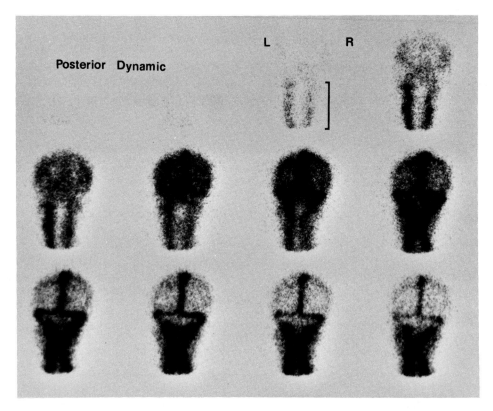

Fig. 10–1. "Flow" (or dynamic) phase of brain study performed with 20 mCi ^{99m}Tc-gluceptate and with patient in posterior position. Initial flow images show decreased delivery of radiopharmaceutical occurring in the right neck vessels (bracketed). Otherwise, the study appears normal.

ment and distribution of the appropriate radiopharmaceutical reflects bulk flow of the CSF. Since several types of disorders alter CSF dynamics, CSF imaging can be valuable in determining specific types of abnormalities.

Principle

Following lumbar subarachnoid injection of the appropriate radiopharmaceutical, sequential scintillation images of radiopharmaceutical migration depict CSF movement through the subarachnoid space. Under normal conditions, radiopharmaceuticals administered into the subarachnoid space will migrate towards the head, reaching the superior sagittal sinus approximately 24 hours after injection. Radiopharmaceuticals must be sufficiently nondiffusible if they are to be confined to the CSF over the imaging interval and should be nonirritating to avoid reactions and side effects.

Indications

CSF imaging is most widely employed to detect and distinguish between two types of hydrocephalus: communicating hydrocephalus and hydrocephalus resulting from cerebral atrophy. Although nuclear medicine CSF imaging has been used less and less since the introduction of CT imaging, it is still useful as a diagnostic aid in the evaluation of the patency of surgical CSF ventricular shunts and can be used to localize CSF leaks.

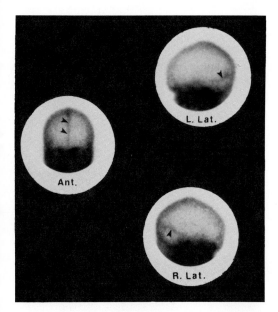

Fig. 10–2. Static study brain image in patient with no evidence of cerebral disorder. *Arrows* indicate normal appearance of blood sinuses. Blood background activity can also be seen around mouth and nasal areas.

Radiopharmaceutical Data

Several radiopharmaceuticals have been employed for CSF imaging, including radioiodinated (I-131) human serum albumin

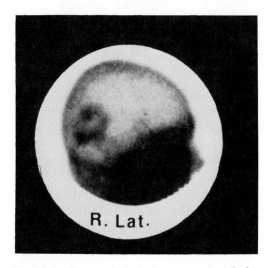

Fig. 10–3. Primary brain lesion as seen in right lateral view. The tumor has a necrotic center, which accounts for the "doughnut" appearance (high uptake around the tumor with no uptake in tumor center).

(RISA), ⁹⁹mTc-DTPA and human serum albumin, ¹¹¹In-DTPA, and ¹⁶⁹Yb-DTPA. Presently, only ¹¹¹In-DTPA and ¹⁶⁹Yb-DTPA are approved for this indication (Table 10–4).

Yb-169 DTPA. This agent has the disadvantages of having a relatively long physical half-life (32 days) and only moderately abundant multiple gamma photon emissions.

Under normal circumstances, the absorbed radiation dose to the brain and spinal cord following administration of the usual adult dose of 500 μCi is approximately 8 rads. With impaired CSF absorption, however, the radiation dose may be substantially increased.

In-111 DTPA. The superior nuclear properties of In-111 makes ¹¹¹In-DTPA the agent of choice for studies of the cerebral spinal fluid kinetics (Table 10–4).

Following a lumbar injection of ¹¹¹In-DTPA the radiopharmaceutical normally migrates to the base of the brain (cisterna magna) in 2 to 3 hours. The agent then passes laterally, ascending symmetrically in front of and along the sides of both cerebral hemispheres (Fig. 10–4). At 24 hours, the radiopharmaceutical flow reaches the superior sagittal sinus.

Abnormal flow patterns include prolonged entry of the radiopharmaceutical into the ventricles and asymmetric, flow patterns or blockage of flow at any level.

Eventually, the radiopharmaceutical is absorbed into venous blood at arachnoid villi and subsequently excreted by the kidneys.

Special Considerations/Patient Preparation

No special patient preparation is necessary.

Methods

Radiopharmaceuticals are injected intrathecally into the lumbar subarachnoid

Table 10–4. Comparison of nuclear properties of radionuclide cisternography agents Yb-169 DTPA and In-111 DTPA.

	Yb-169 DTPA	In-111 DTPA
Physical Half-life	32 days	2.7 days
Principal Photon Energies/Abundance	177 KeV (22%) 198 KeV (35%)	173 KeV (89%) 247 KeV (94%)
Decay Mode	EC	EC
Activity Administered	500 μCi	500 μCi
Radiation Dose to Spinal Cord (500 μCi)	8 rads	1.9 rads

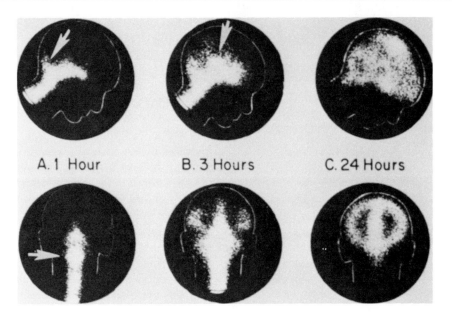

Fig. 10–4. Normal cisternogram showing right lateral (top) and posterior views. At 1 hr, the cisterna magna *(arrows)* and basal cisterns are filled. By 3 hr, the larger quadrigeminal cistern *(arrow)* is visible and activity is entering the sylvan fissures. By 24 hr, activity is distributed completely over the convexities and has largely cleared from the basal cisterns. (From Harbert, JC, Rocha, AFG, (eds.): Textbook of Nuclear Medicine: Clinical Applications, Philadelphia, Lea & Febiger, 1979, p. 88.)

space and images are obtained approximately 4 and 24 hours later. Additional images may be necessary at 48 hours or longer if, at 24 hours, radiopharmaceutical ascent into the parasagittal region is incomplete or if activity remains in the ventricles.

Patient studies for CSF leaks (such as CSF rhinorrhea) may include imaging at 1 to 2 hours postinjection, since CSF flow in these patients is greatly increased and radiopharmaceutical exist from the CSF occurs earlier. The use of nasal packs (pledgets), which are inserted after injection and subsequently assayed for radioactivity in a well-type radiation detector, may be helpful in confirming the presence of CSF rhinorrhea.

REFERENCES

1. Deland, FH, James, AE Jr, Wagner, HN Jr, et al.: Cisternography with [169]Yb-DTPA. J Nucl Med 12:683–689, 1971.

2. Gallagher, BM, Fowler, JS, Gutterson, NI, et al.: Metabolic trapping as a principle of radiopharmaceutical design: Some factors responsible for the biodistribution of [^{18}F] 2-deoxy-2-fluoro-D-glucose. J Nucl Med 19:1154–1161, 1978.

3. Goodwin, DA, Song, CH, Finston, R, et al.: Preparation, physiology and dosimetry of ^{111}In-labeled radiopharmaceuticals for cisternography. Radiology 108:91–98, 1973.

4. Holman, BL, Lee, RGL, Hill, TC, et al.: A comparison of two cerebral perfusion tracers, N-isopropyl I-123 p-Iodoamphetamine and I-123 HIPDM, in the human. J Nucl Med 25:25–30, 1984.

5. Maynard, CD, Cowan, RJ: Static dynamic imaging of the brain. CRC Crit Rev Clin Rad Nucl Med 5:447–477, 1974.

6. Oldendorf, WH: Permeability of the blood brain barrier. In The Nervous System, Vol. I. The Basic Neurosciences. Edited by DB Tower. New York, Raven Press, 1975, pp. 279–289.

7. Ramsey, RG, Quinn, JL III: Comparison of accuracy between initial and delayed ^{99m}Tc-pertechnetate brain scans. J Nucl Med 13:131–134, 1972.

8. Rollo, FD, Vavalieri, RR, Born, M, et al.: Comparative evaluation of Tc-99m-GH, Tc-99m-04, and Tc-99m-DTPA as brain imaging agents. Radiology 123:379–383, 1977.

9. Waxman, AD, Tanasescu, D, Siemsen, JK, et al.: Technetium-99m glucoheptonate as a brain scanning agent: critical comparison with pertechnetate. J Nucl Med 17:345–348, 1976.

10. Witcofski, RL, Janeway, R, Maynard, CD, et al.: Visualization of the choroid plexus on the technetium-99m brain scan. Clinical significance and blocking by potassium perchlorate. Arch Neur 16:286–291, 1967.

11. Wolfstein, RS, Tanasescu, D, Sakimura, IT, et al.: Brain imaging with ^{99m}Tc-DTPA: A clinical comparison of early and delayed studies. J Nucl Med 15:1135–1137, 1974.

11

Radiopharmaceuticals for Thyroid and Adrenal Gland Imaging

11.1 THYROID GLAND FUNCTION

The primary function of the thyroid gland is to regulate the basal metabolic rate by controlling the rate of synthesis and the release of the thyroid hormones, triiodothyronine (T_3) and thyroxine (T_4). These hormones, which are essential to metabolic processes, are synthesized in the thyroid gland by the trapping of iodide from blood, its subsequent oxidation to iodine, and the organification and condensation of these compounds to form T_3 and T_4. Finally, thyroid hormone is stored in the thyroid follicle associated with thyroglobulins.

The synthesis and secretion of thyroid hormone is regulated by thyroid stimulating hormone (TSH), a polypeptide hormone that is secreted by the anterior pituitary. TSH secretion is stimulated by thyrotropin releasing hormone, TRH. Currently, TRH stimulation of the thyroid is considered to be relatively constant. The amount of TSH secreted by the pituitary in response to a constant TRH stimulus is determined largely by the circulating levels of T_4 and T_3. High levels of circulating thyroid hormone suppress pituitary secretion of TSH, whereas low levels of thyroid hormone enhance TSH secretion.

Although T_4 has some intrinsic metabolic activity, T_3 accounts for most of the daily metabolic activity of the thyroid. In serum, T_4 and T_3 are bound primarily to thyroxine-binding globulin (TBG). The binding affinity of T_3 to TBG is only one thirtieth that of T_4. This weaker binding of T_3 to TBG and T_3's greater affinity than T_4 for cellular receptors of the pituitary and other tissues probably accounts for its greater metabolic potency and more rapid turnover in serum. The average plasma half-life for T_3 is approximately 1 day, and that of T_4, approximately 6 days.

Although the thyroid gland is relatively small (normally weighing 20 to 35 grams), its function has a remarkable impact upon the body's metabolic behavior. For example, in *hyperthyroidism*, which is a hypermetabolic state secondary to excessive levels of circulating thyroid hormones, patients have classical symptoms that include extreme nervousness, fatigue, weight loss, and heat intolerance. Hyperthyroidism may result from a variety of clinical disorders, including diffuse toxic goiter (Graves' disease), toxic multinodular goiter, toxic adenoma, subacute thyroiditis, and iodide-induced hyperthyroidism. In Graves' disease, one of the more commonly occurring types of hyperthyroidism, the cause of hyperthyroidism may involve the action of a long-acting thyroid stimulating substance (LATS).

On the other hand, patients with *hypothyroidism* have low levels of circulating thyroid hormones and present with signs and symptoms of hypometabolism including lethargy, cold intolerance, and a tendency to gain weight. In hypothyroid patients, except those with pituitary failure, increased serum levels of thyroid-stimulating hormone are found. Causes of hypothyroidism include an inherited enzyme defect in which physical and mental growth and development are retarded, dietary iodide deficiency, and chronic thyroiditis that is usually of an autoimmune origin. Exogenous thyroid hormone replacement is usually sufficient therapy for hypothyroidism. Myxedema, the end stage of untreated hypothyroidism, manifests as skin changes involving swelling, particularly of the face.

11.2 NUCLEAR MEDICINE STUDIES OF THE THYROID GLAND

When artificially produced radionuclides were initially made available in the late 1930s, radioactive iodine was one of the first to be produced in sizable quantities. At that time a great deal was already known about iodine metabolism, including the fact that large amounts of iodine tended to accumulate in the thyroid gland. The application of radioactive iodine (in particular I-131) to diagnosis and therapy of thyroid gland disorders became apparent, and in the years that followed the use of I-131 for the study of thyroid function grew steadily.

Today, studies of the thyroid gland are not limited to the use of I-131; other radioisotopes of iodine are also available. Additionally, a noniodine radionuclide, ^{99m}Tc-sodium pertechnetate, mimics most of the biological properties of iodine (except organification into thyroid hormone) and is also useful for studying the thyroid gland.

Nuclear medicine studies of the thyroid gland can be classified according to the type of diagnostic information sought. *Thyroid uptake* studies measure gland function by determining the fraction of radioiodine activity taken up by the thyroid gland. *Thyroid imaging* procedures provide visualization of thyroid size, shape, and location and can be performed with either I-123,

I-131 sodium iodide, or ^{99m}Tc-sodium pertechnetate.

11.3 THYROID UPTAKE STUDIES

Principle

Thyroid uptake measurements are based on the thyroid gland's use of iodine in the production of thyroid hormone and the fact that radioactive iodine follows the same metabolic pathways as normally occurring stable iodine (I-127). Using relatively small doses of radioiodine (compared to the total body pool of stable iodine), the fraction of radioiodine taken up by the thyroid can be determined over selected time intervals and compared to known euthyroid values.

Indication

Thyroid uptake measurements are useful in evaluating the function of the thyroid gland, determining the avidity of the gland for iodine prior to therapy, and determining the effect of antithyroid medications.

Radiopharmaceutical Data

Small amounts of I-131 and I-123 (as the sodium iodide salt) may be administered orally in either liquid or capsule form; capsules, however, are usually preferred for accuracy and ease of handling.

Because I-131 has a relatively long physical half-life (8 days) and is a beta emitter, it provides significant radiation dose to the thyroid (Table 11–1) and should be given for thyroid uptake studies in very small quantities (usually 5 to 10 μCi). I-123 on the other hand, because it decays by electron capture and is relatively short-lived (13.0 hr), delivers considerably less thyroidal radiation and can be given for thyroid uptake studies in much higher activities (usually 50 to 100 μCi). With either radiopharmaceutical, the amount of elemental iodide administered is minimal,

Table 11–1.   Radiation dose estimates for I-131 and I-123.

| Radiopharmaceutical | Usual Activity Administered | | Radiation (thyroid) mR/uCi |
	Thyroid Uptake	Thyroid Image	
¹³¹I-sodium iodide	5–10 µCi	35–65 µCi	1200
¹²³I-sodium iodide	50–100 µCi	300–400 µCi	10–15*

*Figures are for I-123 produced by the reaction Te-127 (p, 5n) I-123. I-123 can be produced by other methods; however, higher levels of radionuclidic contaminants such as I-125 and I-131 usually result, which produce substantially higher thyroidal irradiation.

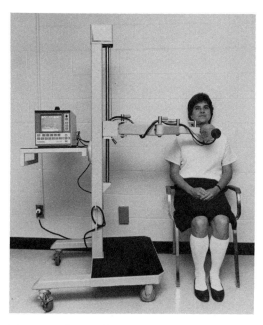

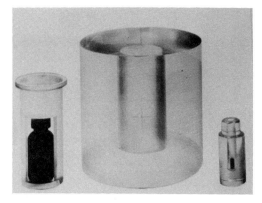

Fig. 11–2. Neck "phantom" for thyroid uptake measurements used to approximate the effect of tissues upon attenuation of gamma emissions. An amount of radioactivity equivalent to that given to the patient is placed into the phantom. Inserts shown (in the left and right of figure) permit phantom to be loaded safely with I-131 in either liquid or capsule form. (Courtesy Atomic Products Corporation.)

Fig. 11–1. Patient shown in position for thyroid uptake measurement. A probe detector is placed against the patient's neck; radioactivity in the thyroid gland is determined as "counts." This information is compared to a standard of radioactivity equivalent to the amount given to the patient.

usually less than 0.0004 µg iodide (the daily adult intake of stable iodide is approximately 150 µg).

Following oral administration, radioactive iodine is absorbed through the intestines and reaches a maximum level in blood within 3 hours. Nearly 90% of the administered dose is excreted in the urine, with less than 2% excreted in feces and perspiration.

Method

The uptake of radioactive iodide by the thyroid gland is expressed as a percentage of the dose administered. This is determined by comparing thyroid activity to a standard that is equivalent to the amount given to the patient. Uptake measurements are usually made at 4 and 24 hours after radioiodide administration and are made using a probe-type sodium iodide [NaI(Tl)] detector with the patient's neck slightly extended (Fig. 11–1). The standard is counted in a simulated neck (known as "phantom") (Fig. 11–2), which mimics the effects of neck tissue upon emitted radiation.

The thyroid uptake is calculated as follows:

$$\text{\% radioiodide uptake} = \frac{A - BKG}{P - BKG} \times 100$$

Table 11–2. Thyroid compartments: approximate values. (Modified from Sadee, W, Finn, C: Stable radionuclides in clinical pharmacology. *In* Radiopharmacy. Edited by M Tubis and W Wolf. New York, John Wiley and Sons, 1976, p. 724.)

Thyroid gland weight: 20 g
Thyroid iodine (trapped iodide and bound iodine): 8000 μg (8 mg)
Trapped iodide concentration: 10–20 μg/100 ml (15 to 50 times the serum concentration)
Trapped iodide pool: less than 10 μg
Extrathyroidal iodine: 1–2 mg
Serum iodide concentration: 0.01–0.41 μg/100 ml
Thyroxine secreted per day: 75–180 μg
Organically bound iodine secreted per day: 50–120 μg
Triiodothyronine secreted per day: 8–20 μg
Radioiodide uptake** at 24 hrs: 27% (Euthyroid)
$\qquad\qquad\qquad\qquad\qquad$ 54% (Hyperthyroid)
$\qquad\qquad\qquad\qquad\qquad$ 5% (Hypothyroid)
Protein-bound iodine (PBI): 6–8 μg/100 ml
Protein-bound thyroxine: (T-4 test): 4–6 μg/100 ml
Free thyroxine (Free T-4): Less than 0.01 μg/100 ml
Binding capacity—Thyroxine-binding globulin (TBG): 20–25 μg/100 ml
$\qquad\qquad\qquad$ Thyroxine-binding prealbumin (TBPA): 250–300 μg/100 ml
$\qquad\qquad\qquad$ Thyroxine-binding albumin: unlimited
Thyroxine bound to TBG*: 50–70% of total thyroxine
Thyroxine bound to prealbumin:* 10%–30% of total thyroxine
Thyroxine bound to albumin:* 5%–20% of total thyroxine
Organically bound iodine secreted per day:* 50–120 μg

*Percentage of thyroxine bound to various components depends on concentration of binding proteins, affinities of components for thyroxine, and concentrations of thyroxine.
**Figures shown represent approximate mean values.

where

A = total counts in patient's thyroid
P = total counts in the thyroid phantom
BKG = background counts

Approximate biological values for the thyroid gland are shown in Table 11–2.

Special Considerations/Patient Preparation

Since thyroid uptake of radioiodide can be affected by alterations in body iodide pool, patients should be carefully screened to ensure that no excessive amount of iodide has been recently ingested or administered. Specifically, materials such as iodinated radiographic contrast agents and iodide-containing expectorants and vitamins suppress iodide uptake by increasing body iodide pool. Other medications can also alter iodide metabolism and influence thyroid uptake of iodide (Table 11–3). To facilitate absorption, oral radioiodine is best administered with the stomach empty.

11.4 THYROID IMAGING

Principle

Radioiodide is trapped and retained by the thyroid, allowing scintillation imaging of the gland (Fig. 11–3). ^{99m}Tc-sodium pertechnetate is also trapped by the thyroid (but not organified) and may be used for thyroid imaging (Fig. 11–4).

Indications

Thyroid imaging is useful in several clinical situations (Table 11–4), such as for determining thyroid size and position and the location and function of thyroid nodules. Hyperfunctioning nodules are generally depicted as areas of increased radiopharmaceutical uptake (Fig. 11–5), while nonfunctioning areas are seen as "cold" regions (Fig. 11–6). Clinically, the significance of "hot" vs "cold" nodules is related to the probability that a nodule harbors cancer. "Hot" nodules are unlikely to be cancerous (incidence less than 1/500), while "cold" thyroid nodules have a much

Table 11–3. Medications known to alter thyroid uptake of radioiodine and ^{99m}Tc-sodium pertechnetate

Depression of Uptake	Duration
Radiographic contrast media	(Depending on specific agent)
—IVP	1–3 wk
—bronchographic	2 mo–2 yr
—myelographic	1+ yr
—gallbladder agents	2+ mo
Exogenous iodides	1–3 wk
—expectorants	
—vitamins	
—topical agents	
Antithyroid medications*	1–2 wk
—propylthiouracil	
—Tapazole^R	
Miscellaneous medications	1+ wk
—salicylates (high doses only)	
—steroids	
—perchlorate	2–3 days
Thyroid hormones	
—Cytomel^R	1–2+ wk
—Synthroid^R	2–4+ wk

*Antithyroid medications only affect radioiodine uptake by the thyroid gland; they have no effect on ^{99m}Tc-sodium pertechnetate.

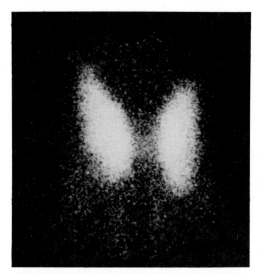

Fig. 11–3. Scintillation images of normal thyroid gland obtained with 400 μCi ^{123}I-sodium iodide.

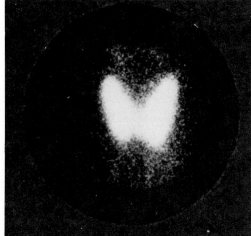

Fig. 11–4. Thyroid image obtained with 10 mCi ^{99m}Tc-sodium pertechnetate. The image appears normal.

Table 11–4.   Indications for thyroid imaging.

1. To determine thyroid size, function, and position.
2. To diagnose thyroid nodules.
3. To differentiate acute thyroiditis from hemorrhage into the gland.
4. To evaluate masses in the lingual region, neck, and mediastinum.

Table 11–5.   Radiopharmaceutical amounts and routes of administration for thyroid imaging.

^{99m}Tc-sodium pertechnetate	5–10 mCi (IV)
^{123}I-sodium iodide	300–400 μCi (PO)
^{131}I-sodium iodide	35–65 μCi (PO)
	1–2 mCi (PO)*

*For whole body imaging in patients with *known* carcinoma.

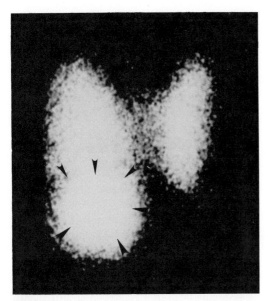

Fig. 11–5.   Thyroid image showing a relatively large hyperfunctioning nodule *(arrows)*.

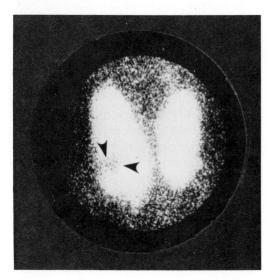

Fig. 11–6.   Thyroid image with a small "cold" nodule *(arrows)*.

greater likelihood of representing cancer (1/5). Rarely, there may be normal trapping of ^{99m}TcO$_4^-$ but absence of radioiodide organification, thus producing a discordant nodule. The incidence of malignancy may be higher with this pattern.

Thyroid imaging is useful in evaluating patients with thyroid carcinoma pre- and postoperatively and in following the effects of therapy on these patients. Whole body imaging with radioiodide is also useful in localizing functioning (iodine-accumulating) metastatic carcinoma.

Radiopharmaceutical Data

As with thyroid uptake studies, either ^{131}I-sodium iodide or ^{123}I-sodium iodide can be used for thyroid imaging. In order to provide adequate count rates for imaging, however, more activity must be administered than that given for thyroid uptake measurements. The activity and route of administration for these agents are shown in Table 11–5. Because of its beta emission and high radiation dose, I-131 is usually reserved for total body surveys for localizing functioning metastatic carcinoma. I-123 has excellent imaging properties, but its relatively short physical half-life (13 hr) limits availability. ^{99m}Tc-sodium pertechnetate is the preferred agent for routine thyroid imaging if I-123 is not available.

Method

With both ^{123}I- and ^{131}I-sodium iodide, patient images are obtained 18 to 24 hours after administration, although earlier imaging is possible. Thyroid imaging with intravenously administered ^{99m}Tc-sodium pertechnetate is best performed 20 to 30 minutes after injection.

Special Considerations/Patient Preparation

Neither orally administered radioiodine nor intravenously administered ^{99m}Tc-sodium pertechnetate requires special patient preparation. Patients should be carefully screened, however, to ensure that they are not taking medications that alter thyroid uptake (Table 11–3).

Interventional Agents

In thyroid imaging, pharmacologic intervention is occasionally desirable in order to improve diagnostic accuracy. In the evaluation of suspected autonomous thyroid nodules, for example, administration of T_3 will diminish radiopharmaceutical uptake in normal tissues yet will have little effect upon uptake in autonomous thyroid nodules. Radiopharmaceutical uptake by the thyroid can also be stimulated. TSH may be administered to increase radiopharmaceutical uptake in previously suppressed thyroid tissue.

11.5 RADIOPHARMACEUTICALS FOR ADRENAL GLAND IMAGING

Diagnostic techniques other than nuclear medicine offer only anatomic observation of the adrenal glands and do not permit evaluation of adrenal gland function. Nuclear medicine procedures permit functional assessment of the adrenal glands using radiopharmaceuticals that localize by specific uptake pathways in either the adrenal cortex or the medulla.

11.6 ADRENAL CORTICAL IMAGING

Principle

Cholesterol is utilized within the adrenal cortex (and other tissue of mammals) as a substrate for the synthesis of steroid hormones. Attempts to prepare a suitable radiolabeled cholesterol that would maintain the normal distribution of cholesterol (and thus be useful for adrenal imaging) were largely unsuccessful until 1970, when 19-^{131}I-iodocholesterol was synthesized.

Indications

Adrenal cortical imaging is a valuable study in Cushing's syndrome and primary aldosteronism for distinguishing unilateral adenoma from bilateral adrenal hyperplasia.

Radiopharmaceutical Data

During the original research of ^{131}I-19-iodocholesterol, a radiochemical impurity noted in this radiopharmaceutical was subsequently isolated and identified as ^{131}I-NP-59, or 6β-^{131}I-iodomethyl-19-normethylcholesterol (Fig. 11–7). Animal tissue distribution studies revealed that uptake of this compound by the adrenal cortex was 5 to 10 times greater than that of ^{131}I-19-iodocholesterol, with adrenal cortex to liver and kidney ratios as high as 100 noted five days after injection.

The estimated patient radiation dose to the adrenals following intravenous administration of 1 mCi of ^{131}I-NP-59 is relatively high compared to most other nuclear medicine diagnostic studies (extrapolated from animal tissue distribution data to be 150 rads and calculated to be approximately 25 rads from measurements of activity in human tissue excised at surgery).

Method

The adult dose is 1 to 1.5 mCi of ^{131}I-NP-59 administered slowly by the intravenous

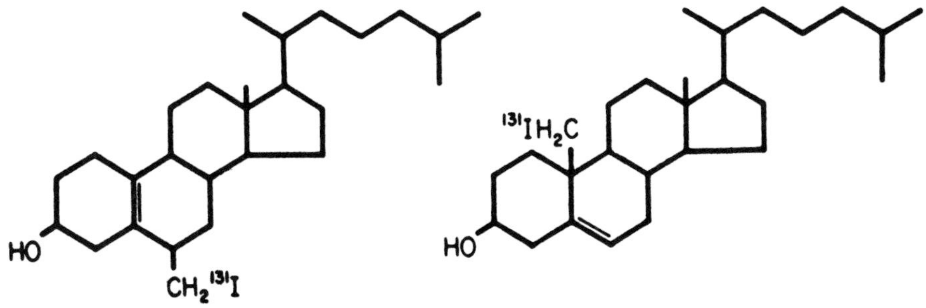

^{131}I-NP-59

(6β-^{131}I-IODOMETHYL-19-NORMETHYL-CHOLESTEROL 5(10)-EN-3β-OL)

^{131}I-19-IODOCHOLESTEROL

(^{131}I-19-IODOCHOLEST-5(6)-EN-3β-OL)

Fig. 11–7. Structures of the adrenal imaging agents ^{131}I-NP-59 (left) and ^{131}I-19-iodocholesterol (right). (Taken from Rocha, AFG, Harbert, JC: Textbook on nuclear medicine: Clinical Applications. Philadelphia, Lea & Febiger, 1979, p. 376.)

route (usually over 3 to 5 minutes). Since the adrenal-to-background count rate ratios improve over a period of several days following administration (because of blood clearance), imaging may necessarily extend to two, three, or four days in order to obtain satisfactory adrenal images.

In patients suspected of aldosterone-producing neoplasms, steroid suppression by the concomitant administration of dexamethasone (Decadron) is advisable. Dexamethasone will suppress ^{131}I-NP-59 uptake by normal adrenal tissues but not by aldosterone-producing tumors.

Special Considerations/Patient Preparation

To prevent thyroidal irradiation from free (unbound) I-131, patients should be pretreated with stable iodide starting one day prior to ^{131}I-NP-59 administration and continuing for 1 to 2 weeks thereafter (Table 11–6).

Table 11–6. Prevention of radioiodine uptake by thyroid gland (thyroid blockade).

1. *Pharmaceuticals*
   Lugol's solution (Strong Iodide Solution, USP)
   Contains, in each 100 ml
   4.5 to 5.5 g iodide, and
   9.5 to 10.5 g potassium iodide
   Saturated Solution Potassium Iodide (SSKI)
   (Potassium Iodide Solution NF)
   Contains, in each 100 ml
   97.0 to 103 g potassium iodide

2. *Procedure for Thyroid Blockade*
   Because of its higher iodide concentration, SSKI is generally preferred for thyroid blockade. Lugol's solution can and is being used; however, large amounts of Lugol's solution must be given in order to ensure adequate blockade of radioiodine uptake by the thyroid gland.
   DOSAGE: Give patient 5 drops SSKI 24 hours prior to administration of radiopharmaceutical, then 3 to 5 drops SSKI b.i.d. for 1 to 2 weeks following radiopharmaceutical administration.

11.7 RADIOPHARMACEUTICALS FOR ADRENAL MEDULLARY IMAGING

The adrenal medulla is a specialized ganglia of sympathetic cells that secrete the biologically active catecholamines epinephrine and norepinephrine. Researchers have attempted to study the adrenal medulla, as well as the heart, another organ with higher levels of the sympathetic neurotransmitters, using radiolabeled epinephrine and norepinephrine. Unfortunately, only radiocarbon-labeled

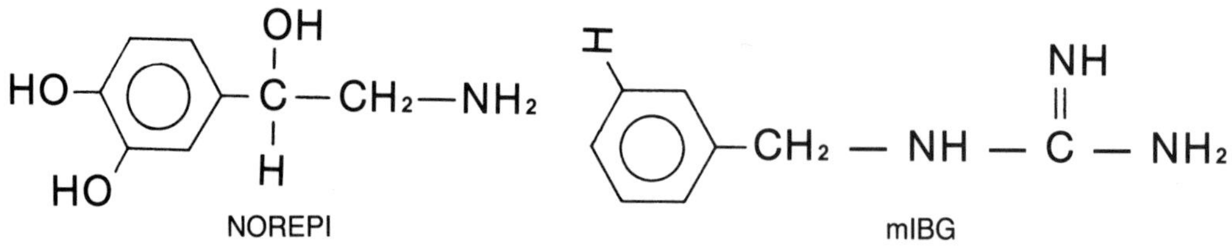

Fig. 11–8. Chemical structures of norepinephrine (NOREPI) and radioiodinated metaiodobenzylguanidine (mIBG).

derivatives of these substances have been prepared, and no gamma-emitting radio-isotope of carbon exists that is suitable for routine use in medicine.

The recent development of meta-[131I]-io-dobenzylguanidine (131I-mIBG), an analogue of the adrenergic blocking agent guanethidine, appears to have the same uptake and storage mechanisms as norepinephrine (Fig. 11–8). 131I-mIBG, however, is not metabolized by either monoamine oxidase or catechol-o-methyl transferase.

Indications

The primary indication for adrenal medullary imaging is the detection of pheochromocytoma.

Radiopharmaceutical Data

Currently, meta-[131I]-iodobenzylguanidine is an investigational agent available for use only by qualified investigators at a limited number of institutions.

REFERENCES

1. Beirwaltes, WH, Wieland, DM, Yu, T, et al.: Adrenal imaging agents: rationale, synthesis, formulation and metabolism. Semin Nucl Med 8:5–22, 1978.
2. Gross, MD, Valk, TW, Swanson, DP, et al.: The role of pharmacologic manipulation in adrenal cortical scintigraphy. Semin Nucl Med 11:128–148, 1981.
3. Keyes, JW, Thrall, JH, Carey, JE: Technical considerations in in vivo thyroid studies. Semin Nucl Med 8:43–58, 1978.
4. Wellman, HN, Kereiakes, JG, Branson, BM: Total and partial-body counting of children for radiopharmaceutical dosimetry data. In Medical Radionuclides: Radiation Dose and Effects. Edited by RL Coutier, CL Edwards, WS Snyder. Springfield, VA, AEC Symposium Series 20 (National Technical Information Service), p. 133, 1970.

CHAPTER

12

Radiopharmaceuticals for Gastrointestinal Imaging

12.1 LIVER IMAGING

The liver, which is the largest organ (approximately 5% of body weight), consists of several lobes, each of which is divided into lobules. Within the lobules are vascular sinusoids whose walls consist of two types of cells: (1) the hepatocytes (or polygonal cells), which carry out the liver's metabolic and excretory functions, and (2) Kupffer's (or reticuloendothelial) cells. Nuclear medicine studies of the liver are classified according to which liver cell type is utilized for radiopharmaceutical uptake. Studies involving hepatocyte function (hepatobiliary) will be discussed first.

12.2 HEPATOBILIARY IMAGING AND HEPATOCYTES

Principle

One of the many metabolic processes performed by the hepatocytes is the initiation of bile formation. Bile, which is composed of red blood cell breakdown products (such as heme and bilirubin), is secreted from the liver via the hepatic duct into the gallbladder. In the gallbladder, bile is concentrated and stored for later discharge through the cystic duct into the common bile duct and into the intestines (Fig. 12–1). Noninvasive studies of hepatocellular function (including studies of biliary tract obstruction) are performed using radiopharmaceuticals that are taken up by hep-

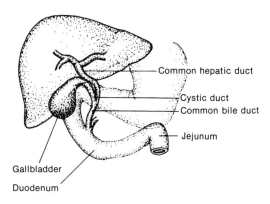

Fig. 12–1. Liver anatomy, including biliary system.

atocytes through active transport mechanisms and excreted via the hepatobiliary pathway into the intestines.

Indications

Hepatobiliary imaging is useful in the diagnosis of acute cholecystitis and in the differentiation of jaundice resulting from hepatocellular causes from jaundice resulting from partial or complete biliary obstruction (although hepatobiliary imaging will not allow absolute differentiation of these two causes). It is also indicated in the evaluation of infants suspected of biliary atresia.

Radiopharmaceutical Data

Until recently, ^{131}I-rose bengal, a triphenylmethane dye extracted from blood by the polygonal cells, was the primary radiopharmaceutical for hepatobiliary imaging. ^{131}I-rose bengal is far from ideal be-

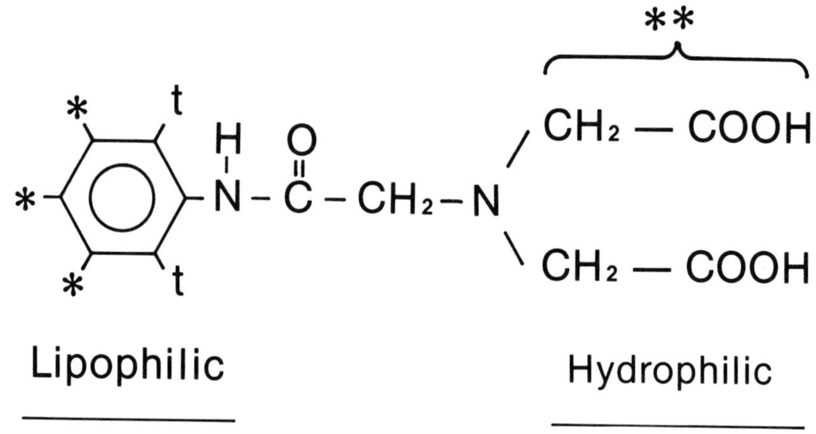
**
*
t
H O
N - C - CH2 - N
CH2 — COOH
CH2 — COOH
Lipophilic
Hydrophilic

Site of Chemical Alteration	Effect
*	Protein Binding
t	Hepatic Kinetics
**	Ability to Chelate Tc-99m

Fig. 12–2. Basic chemical structure of IDA agents used for hepatobiliary imaging, and the effect of chemical substitution upon liver pharmacokinetics. (Note—for uniformity in nomenclature the suffix *-fenin* is now used to denote compounds of the basic IDA-type structure, e.g., lido*fenin*, etc.)

NAME	R_1	R_2	R_3	R_4
Butilfenin	–H	$-CH_2(CH_2)_2CH_3$	–H	–H
Disofenin	$-CH(CH_3)_2$	–H	–H	$-CH(CH_3)_2$
Etifenin	$-C_2H_5$	–H	–H	$-C_2H_5$
Lidofenin (HIDA)	$-CH_3$	–H	–H	$-CH_3$
Mebrofenin	$-CH_3$	$-CH_3$	–Br	$-CH_3$

*From USAN 1986: USAN and the USP dictionary of drug names.

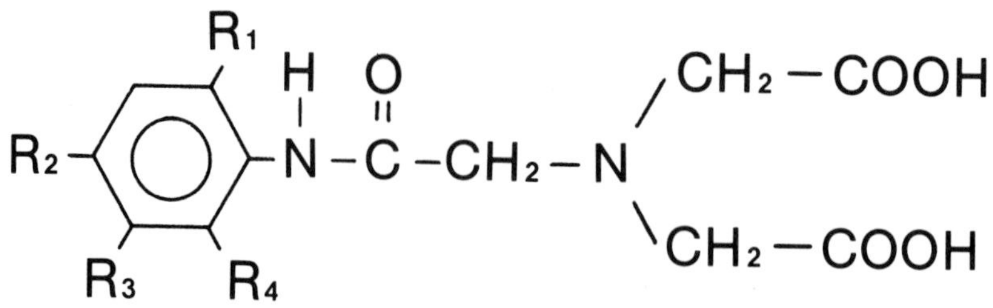
R1
R2
R3
R4
H O
N - C - CH2 - N
CH2 - COOH
CH2 - COOH

Fig. 12–3. Selected IDA-type agents and their chemical structures.*

cause of its poor imaging characteristics, its high patient radiation dose with limited activity administered, and its extrahepatic excretion, which occurs in moderate-to-severe liver disease.[131]I-rose bengal has recently been replaced by the Tc-99m–labeled derivatives of iminodiacetic acid (IDA).

The IDA-type radiopharmaceuticals are called "bifunctional" because they possess both a hydrophilic group necessary for binding Tc-99m and a lipophilic component that provides hepatocellular specificity (Fig. 12–2). It is possible to alter basic pharmacodynamic properties by substituting onto the phenyl (lipophilic) ring groups that increase overall lipophilicity or decrease protein binding. The chemical structures of several of these derivatives and that of lidofenin (or HIDA), the early prototype of this group of agents, is shown in Fig. 12–3. Experimental studies have shown that these Tc-99m compounds probably exist as dimers, with two molecules of the IDA derivative bound by a central atom of Tc-99m (Fig. 12–4).

Tc-99m disofenin, a commonly used Tc-99m–labeled IDA derivative, is rapidly cleared from the blood of normal patients, with about only 8% of the dose remaining 30 minutes following injection. In patients with normal liver function, less than 8% of the injected dose is excreted in the urine over the first two hours (higher amounts, however, may be excreted in urine of patients with impaired liver function).

The upper large intestines receive approximately 2 rads from the usual 5 mCi adult dose of ^{99m}Tc-disofenin.

Method

In nonjaundiced adult patients the usual dose of ^{99m}Tc-disofenin is 3 to 5 mCi; however, patients with serum bilirubin levels greater than 5 mg/dl may be given as much as 10 mCi in order to adequately visualize the biliary pathway. Scintillation imaging is begun soon after radiopharmaceutical administration, with images obtained serially at intervals of 5 to 15 minutes. In fasting normal subjects, peak liver uptake of the radiopharmaceutical usually occurs by 10 minutes after injection, with maximum gallbladder accumulation at 30 to 40 minutes (Fig. 12–5). In normal individuals visualization of gallbladder and intestinal activity should occur by 60 minutes after injection. If the gallbladder and intestines are visualized the study is complete. If either organ is not visualized by 60 mintues, delayed images at hourly intervals may be obtained for up to 24 hours, if necessary.

Special Considerations/Patient Preparation

Patients should fast for at least four hours prior to injection since false positive studies may result if the gallbladder has been emptied by the ingestion of food.

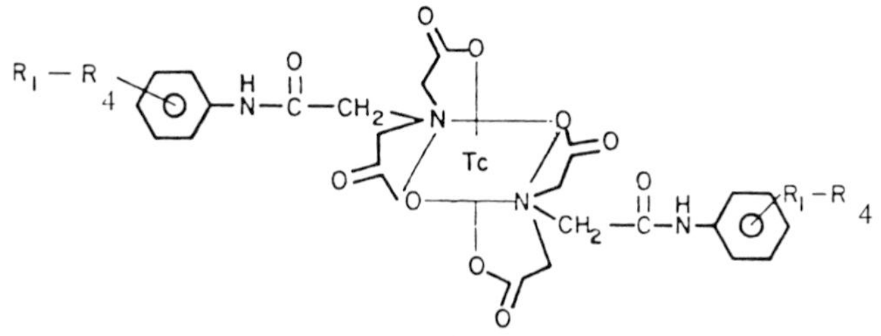

Fig. 12–4. Proposed structure of ^{99m}Tc-lidofenin. (From Nunn, AD, Loberg, MD: Hepatobiliary agents. In Radiopharmaceuticals: Structure-Activity Relationships. Edited by RP Spencer. New York, Grune and Stratton, 1981, pp. 539–548, by permission.)

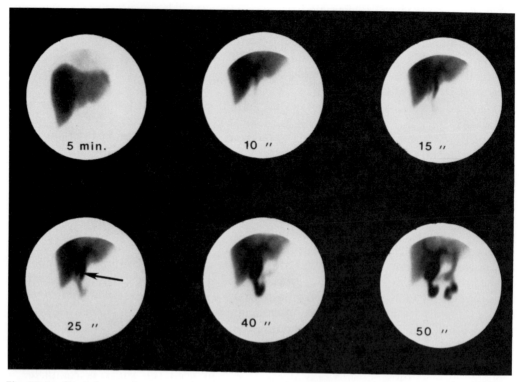

Fig. 12–5. Scintiphotos taken up to 50 minutes after administration of ^{99m}Tc-disofenin. Note gallbladder *(arrow)* and intestinal activity.

studies may result if the gallbladder has been emptied by the ingestion of food.

12.3 ARCHITECTURAL LIVER IMAGING (KUPFFER'S CELLS)

Principle

The Kupffer's cells are the primary cells of the reticuloendothelial (RE) system and are located throughout healthy liver tissue, in the spleen, and in the bone marrow. The RE system removes foreign matter from blood by phagocytosis.

In normal individuals, approximately 85% of the RE cells are located in the liver, 10% in the spleen, and the remaining 5% in bone marrow. When radiolabeled particles, called colloids, are injected intravenously, they will be phagocytized by these RE cells, and scintillation images of liver and spleen in normal individuals show ho-

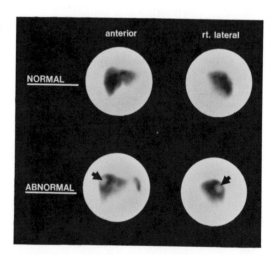

Fig. 12–6. Scintiphotos taken in anterior and right lateral positions of patients injected with ^{99m}Tc-sulfur colloid. In normal patients, the radiopharmaceutical distributes uniformly in the liver and spleen. In patients with disease that disrupts normal Kupffer's cell function, the involved area is shown as a "cold" region *(arrows)* that fails to localize this radiopharmaceutical.

Table 12–1. Indications for radiocolloid liver imaging.

1. To evaluate liver size, shape, and position
2. To detect focal space-occupying lesions such as tumors, cysts, and abscesses
3. To evaluate abdominal masses
4. To evaluate preoperative hepatic metastasis in patients with known malignancies
5. To localize hepatic lesions for biopsy or of abscesses for drainage
6. To follow up patients with liver metastasis undergoing chemotherapy or radiation therapy
7. To work up patients with diffuse hepatic disease, such as cirrhosis or hepatitis

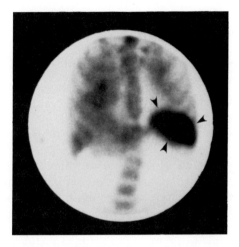

Fig. 12–7. Scintiphoto (anterior) of patient injected with ^{99m}Tc-sulfur colloid showing "colloid shift." Note the visualization of the spleen *(arrows)* and bone marrow activity. The liver has only slight uptake and is faintly visualized.

mogeneous distribution of the radioactive colloid throughout these organs (Fig. 12–6). Areas affected by disease, on the other hand, fail to localize this radiopharmaceutical. Presently, the most commonly employed radiocolloid is ^{99m}Tc-sulfur colloid.

Indications

Architectural liver imaging has several indications (Table 12–1).

Radiopharmaceutical Data

Tc-99m Sulfur Colloid. This radiopharmaceutical is prepared from commercially available kits (Chapter 8) and generator-produced ^{99m}Tc-sodium pertechnetate.

Following intravenous administration, the biological half-life of ^{99m}Tc-sulfur colloid in blood is approximately 3 minutes. In normal patients, 80 to 85% of the injected dose localizes in liver, 5 to 10% in spleen, and the remainder primarily in bone marrow. In severe hepatic disease, increased amounts of ^{99m}Tc-sulfur colloid may be taken up by the RE cells of the spleen and bone marrow ("colloid shift") (Fig. 12–7). Inorganic particulate matter (including ^{99m}Tc-sulfur colloid) is not metabolized by the cells of the RE system and becomes "fixed" indefinitely in the Kupffer's cells following phagocytosis. To date, however, no adverse effects have been noted from this long-term retention.

Tc-99m Microaggregated Albumin. Another radiopharmaceutical useful for architectural liver imging is ^{99m}Tc-microaggregated albumin. This radiopharmaceutical is prepared by the microaggregation of human serum albumin and uses the stannous ion reduction method for Tc-99m radiolabeling. ^{99m}Tc-microaggregated albumin has approximately the same biological distribution in the reticuloendothelial system as ^{99m}Tc-sulfur colloid. Radiopharmaceutical uptake in the liver and spleen is essentially complete by 15 minutes after injection and remains constant for at least four hours thereafter. Unlike ^{99m}Tc-sulfur colloid, however, ^{99m}Tc-microaggregated albumin is cleared from the liver by metabolic activity.

With either ^{99m}Tc-sulfur colloid or ^{99m}Tc-microaggregated albumin, the critical organ is the liver, which receives approximately 0.3 rads/mCi.

Method

Patients are injected with 3 to 5 mCi of either ^{99m}Tc-sulfur colloid or ^{99m}Tc-microaggregated albumin, and static images are taken approximately 15 mintues later. Scintiphotos of liver and spleen are usually obtained in at least four views.

Special Considerations/Patient Preparation

No special patient preparation is necessary.

Generator eluate containing more than 10 μg Al^{+3}/ml should not be used in the preparation of ^{99m}Tc-sulfur colloid, since aluminum ions cause flocculation of this radiopharmaceutical, resulting in the formation of larger colloidal particles, which would be taken up by the lungs rather than by the liver. The actual mechanism involves alteration by electropositive aluminum ions of the usually highly electronegative zeta potential, which acts to stabilize the colloid particle size (the colorimetric test for aluminum ions in generator eluate is discussed in Chapter 9). Aluminum interference with colloid size, however, is not limited to in vitro situations; hyperaluminemia secondary to large-volume aluminum hydroxide therapy has also been reported to cause in vivo flocculation of ^{99m}Tc-sulfur colloid and subsequent increased lung uptake.

The on-site preparation of ^{99m}Tc-sulfur colloid requires heating (i.e., in a boiling water bath) following the addition of generator-produced Tc-99m sodium pertechnetate. Usually the suggested heating time is 5 to 12 minutes (depending upon product formulation). Heating times should be carefully monitored since it is known that heating prolonged beyond the manufacturer's specified time can be another cause of undesirably large colloid particles.

Tc-99m microaggregated albumin does not require heating during on-site preparation.

12.4 OTHER GASTROINTESTINAL IMAGING PROCEDURES

Spleen Imaging

Occasionally, it is desirable to visualize only the spleen, without interfering liver or bone marrow activity. This type of situation arises when attempting to locate accessory splenic tissues in patients with continued evidence of hypersplenism after splenectomy. Since the spleen is the site of sequestration of senescent red blood cells, radiolabeled autologous red blood cells that have been heat-damaged will also be sequestered by the spleen. No uptake in liver or bone marrow occurs when the labeled red cells are properly prepared.

In spite of its relatively poor imaging properties, Cr-51 (as sodium chromate) was for many years the only suitable agent available for red blood cell labeling. Recently, techniques for red cell labeling with Tc-99m have been developed. Spleen imaging can be performed using RBCs that are labeled with Tc-99m (using the Sn^{+2} labeling process) and heat damaged. The temperature used to damage the red cells is critical, since inadequately damaged cells will not be sequestered by the spleen, and severely damaged cells will localize in *both* the liver and the spleen.

Pancreas Imaging

For many years ^{75}Se-selenomethionine, a radiolabeled amino acid analogue utilized just like methionine in the synthesis of digestive enzymes, had been the only radiopharmaceutical routinely available for pancreas imaging. Generally, pancreas imaging with this agent has been disappointing because of the variable shape and size of the pancreas and the poor radiopharmaceutical uptake characteristics (less than 7% of the injected dose localizes in the pancreas). Further, concentration of the radiopharmaceutical in the liver and small intestines, coupled with the slow biological clearance and long physical half-life, subjects the liver and kidney to approximately 6.0 rads from 250 μCi of ^{75}Se-selenomethionine. Other imaging modalities such as CT and ultrasound provide superior images of the pancreas and have made pancreas imaging with ^{75}Se-selenomethionine practically obsolete.

Studies of Gastric Function

Gastric Emptying. Scintigraphic solid-phase gastric emptying measurements, performed either alone or in combination with liquid-phase measurements, are useful in investigating several autonomic gastric neuropathies and evaluating gastric function following surgical procedures. While liquid-phase gastric emptying studies can be easily performed with any of several well-known radiopharmaceuticals (e.g., ^{99m}Tc-DTPA, ^{111}In-DTPA, etc.), solid-phase studies require more-complicated marker preparation involving incorporation of a radionuclide into a suitable solid meal. For example, the "gold standard" solid-phase marker, in vivo intracellular-labeled chicken liver, is prepared by intravenously injecting a live chicken with ^{99m}Tc-sulfur colloid, killing the chicken, and removing and cooking the liver. Because this is an awkward and time-consuming process, in vitro–labeled chicken liver is the preferred agent. This marker is prepared by injecting ^{99m}Tc-sulfur colloid into a chicken liver at multiple sites, then cooking the liver and mixing it into beef stew or another suitable food.

Following patient consumption of the radiolabeled food, computer-assisted imaging techniques measure the time required for stomach emptying. These measurements are compared to those of normal, healthy individuals.

Esophageal Transit. Studies of esophageal transit are performed using a water-insoluble radiopharmaceutical, such as ^{99m}Tc-sulfur colloid. The radiopharmaceutical is administered orally, usually in half an ounce of water, and the passage of the bolus is depicted scintigraphically and quantified by computer assistance. The time necessary to clear 90% of activity from the entire esophagus is measured (areas of interest may also be drawn over each third

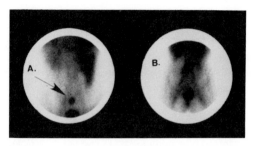

Fig. 12–8. Patient with Meckel's diverticulum *(arrow)* (Image A) and patient with normal distribution of ^{99m}Tc-sodium pertechnetate (Image B). Both images were obtained in the anterior position approximately 10 minutes following intravenous administration of ^{99m}Tc-sodium pertechnetate.

of the esophagus to locate the region of greatest abnormality) and compared to normal values. Solid phase studies of esophageal emptying are especially helpful in severe disease such as stricture or achalasia.

Gastric Mucosa Imaging. Following intravenous administration, ^{99m}Tc-sodium pertechnetate is concentrated and secreted in a variety of tissues, including the thyroid and salivary glands, choroid plexus, and gastric mucosa (including the ectopic gastric mucosa of Meckel's diverticula). Meckel's diverticula will appear as a localized area of increased ^{99m}Tc-sodium pertechnetate uptake (Fig. 12–8) in the right lower quadrant (usually no computer assistance is necessary to adequately image the involved tissues). The normal appearance of the radiopharmaceutical in the stomach and bladder may mask abnormal sites and make visualization of the diverticulum difficult. Patients to be studied should fast for 8 to 12 hours.

REFERENCES

1. Agnew, JE, Maze, M, Mitchell, CJ: Review article: pancreatic scanning. Brit J Rad *49*:979–995, 1976.
2. Berquist, TH, Nolan, NG, Adson, MA, et al.: Diagnosis of Meckel's diverticulum by radioisotope scanning. Mayo Clin Proc *48*:98–102, 1973.
3. Chervu, LR, Nunn, AD, Loberg, MD: Radiopharmaceuticals for hepatobiliary imaging. Semin Nucl Med *12*:5–17, 1982.
4. Gumerman, LW: Nuclear medicine studies in the

diagnosis of the liver, pancreas and spleen. Surg Clin North Am 55:427–447, 1975.

5. Hatfield, PM: Role of liver scanning in the diagnosis of hepatic metastases.: Med Clin North Am 59:247–276, 1975.

6. Kloiber, R, Dawtew, B, Rosenthall, L: A crossover study comparing the effect of particle size on the distribution of radiocolloid in patients. Clin Nucl Med 6:204–206, 1981.

7. Meyer, JH, Bac Gregor, MB, Gueller, R, et al.: Tc-99m tagged chicken liver as a marker of solid food in the human stomach. Digest Dis 21:296–304, 1976.

8. Ryan, J, Cooper, M, Loberg, M, et al.: Technetium 99m labeled N-(2,6-dimethylphenylcarbomoyl-methyl) iminodiactic acid (Tc-99m HIDA): a new radiopharmaceutical for hepatobiliary imaging. J Nucl Med 18:997–1004, 1977.

9. Saba, TM: Physiology and pathophysiology of the reticuloendothelial system. Arch Int Med 126:1031–1052, 1970.

10. Winzelberg, GG, McKusick, KA, Froelich, JW, et al.: Detection of gastrointestinal bleeding with ^{99m}Tc-labeled red blood cells. Semin Nucl Med 12:139–147, 1982.

11. Jarvis, L. Personal communication.

Radiopharmaceuticals for Tumor Detection and Hematologic Studies

13.1 TUMOR DETECTION

The early detection of neoplastic disease has been one of nuclear medicine's major goals. Two approaches to tumor detection have been used.

The first radiopharmaceutical localization mechanism uses some function of the nearby normal tissues that is not shared by the malignant tissues. For example, when the reticuloendothelial system of the liver is studied with Tc-99m sulfur colloid, the tumor is seen as an area of relatively low activity (a so-called cold spot). Agents that use this indirect approach to tumor imaging use organ-specific pathways for radiopharmaceutical uptake and are discussed under the individual organ systems.

Another approach to tumor detection involves the direct visualization of the tumor itself, using as a localization mechanism tumor characteristics not found in normal tissues. With this approach, the tumor is seen as an area of relatively high uptake (i.e., a "hot" spot). Several agents use this approach for tumor detection. Some of the agents in current use (Table 13–1) are specific for one tumor type, whereas other agents are taken up by a wide variety of neoplasms as well as some benign processes. Tumor characteristics that have been utilized as radiopharmaceutical uptake pathways are shown in Table 13–2.

An ideal agent with appropriate tumor specificity and sensitivity and suitable physical decay characteristics has not been found. It appears, however, that at present Ga-67 (as citrate) provides the best overall uptake in most types of tumor and is the preferred agent for routine screening for most soft-tissue tumors.

Table 13–1. Selected radiopharmaceuticals currently used for tumor detection.

Ga-67 citrate
P-32 sodium phosphate
I-131 sodium iodide
I-131 iodocholesterol
Se-75 selenomethionine
Tc-99m diphosphonates

13.2 TUMOR IMAGING WITH ^{67}Ga-CITRATE

Principle

The initial clinical application of radiogallium was for radiation therapy of bone

Table 13–2. Selected tumor characteristics that have been utilized in nuclear medicine as radiopharmaceutical localization pathways.

Increased blood flow to tumor (resulting in greater delivery of tracer to tumor)
Increased metabolic activity whereby radiopharmaceuticals enter tumor cells as metabolic substrates
Altered cellular integrity, permitting entry of radiopharmaceuticals that are normally excluded
Altered intracellular microvasculature, allowing longer extravascular residence time of protein-bound tracers
The presence of tumor-associated antigens that may be detected by radiolabeled antibody.

Table 13–3.   Types of neoplastic and non-neoplastic diseases detected by Ga-67 imaging.

Reliably Detected
   (Neoplastic)
      Hodgkin's disease
      Histiocytic lymphoma
      Acute lymphocytic leukemia
      Acute myelocytic leukemia
      Chronic myelocytic leukemia
      Lung carcinoma
      Hepatoma
      Bone sarcoma

   (Non-Neoplastic)
      Pyogenic abscess
      Sarcoid
      Acute inflammation

Moderately reliably detected
   (Neoplastic)
      Lymphatic lymphoma
      Breast carcinoma
      Epithelial, head, and neck carcinoma
      Gastrointestinal tumor
      Thyroid carcinoma

   (Non-Neoplastic)
      Active tuberculosis

Table 13–4.   Nuclear properties of Ga-67.

$$^{67}Ga \xrightarrow[T^{1/2}p \ = \ 78 \ hr]{EC} {}^{67}Zn \ (stable)$$

Principal Gamma Emissions (KeV)	Yield
93	38%
184	24%
300	16%
393	4%

Indications

^{67}Ga-citrate is useful in demonstrating the presence and extent of soft-tissue tumors, such as Hodgkin's disease, lymphomas, and bronchogenic carcinoma (Table 13–3). As a general rule, Ga-67 detects primary tumors more reliably than it detects metastatic lesions.

Ga-67 concentration also occurs in nonneoplastic lesions such as pyogenic abscesses and focal areas of acute inflammation including osteomyelitis, pneumonia, pyelonephritis, and active tuberculosis. A number of other conditions that cause inflammation or increased blood flow, such as Paget's disease and granulomatous diseases (sarcoidosis), result in increased Ga-67 imaging.

Radiopharmaceutical Data

Gallium is a member of Group III of the periodic chart, which also includes the elements aluminum and indium. Although the element gallium is quite toxic, accelerator-produced Ga-67 contains very little gallium (a patient dose contains less than 10^{-7} mg elemental Ga per kg of human body weight). The nuclear properties of Ga-67 are shown in Table 13–4.

Following administration, about 30% of Ga-67 in blood is bound to plasma proteins, mainly transferrin and to a lesser extent albumin and globulins. The nonprotein-bound fraction diffuses throughout the extravascular space or is excreted by the kidneys. Because of protein binding only about 25% of an injected dose is excreted by the kidneys in the first 24 hours. An-

tumors and used gallium-72, a carrier-containing reactor product. While the primary purpose of that investigation was not achieved, the results demonstrated that the amount of carrier in gallium influenced biological distribution. Specifically, carrier-free radioisotopes of gallium distributed largely in the liver, spleen and kidneys, while carrier-containing Ga-72 showed a greater uptake within the skeleton than in soft tissue. Since carrier-containing Ga-72 has relatively poor nuclear properties (β^- decay with an associated principal photon emission at 835 KeV), carrier-free Ga-67 was subsequently evaluated for use as a bone-scanning agent. It was while scanning the bones of a patient with Hodgkin's disease that ^{67}Ga-citrate uptake by tumor was noted. Ga-67 uptake in selected human and animal tumors has been shown to be very high (as much as 10% of the injected dose per gram of tumor) though some tumor types have failed to show any Ga-67 uptake.

other 10% of the dose is excreted in the stool over the next week (see Special Considerations/Patient Preparation), and the remaining 65% is distributed in the body.

At 2 to 3 days after injection, the highest concentrations of Ga-67 are seen in the liver (5% of administered dose), spleen (1%), kidneys (2%), and skeleton (including marrow, 24%).

To date, several different mechanisms for Ga-67 uptake by tumor have been proposed; the most widely accepted mechanism is shown in Fig. 13–1. The precise mechanism, however, and the reasons for high concentration by some tumors and not by others is not fully understood. Ga-67 uptake in inflammation probably occurs by an entirely different mechanism. One explanation of this uptake mechanism suggests leukocyte labeling by gallium and the migration of these radiolabeled substances to the inflammatory area.

In the spleen, Ga-67 is accumulated in the phagocytic cells, while in the liver both Kupffer's cells and hepatocytes show gallium uptake.

Method

The usual administered activity of ^{67}Ga-citrate for adults is between 3 and 8 mCi given intravenously. Images for tumor detection are obtained at 48 to 72 hours after injection (Fig. 13–2), while images for abscess detection are usually taken at 24 hours.

Ga-67 imaging is usually performed by "peaking" camera windows around the first three principal photopeaks (93, 184, and 300 KeV). The use of a medium energy (high resolution) collimator is preferred.

The normal gallium image shows the greatest accumulation in liver and throughout the skeleton and bone marrow. The spleen may show minimal uptake but frequently is not visualized. Normal variants include Ga-67 uptake in the nasopharynx, lacrimal glands, salivary glands, and external genitalia. Ga-67 uptake has been noted in the human breast and it is secreted in breast milk during pregnancy, lactation, and estrogen therapy. The large bowel is the critical organ and receives a radiation dose of approximately 0.9 rads/mCi.

Special Considerations/Patient Preparation

Since Ga-67 is normally excreted by the bowel, adequate bowel cleansing is necessary before imaging, particularly when the abdomen is a site of a possible disorder.

Previous radiation or chemotherapy may decrease Ga-67 tumor uptake, while surgical wounds can cause increased Ga-67 localization for several weeks afterwards.

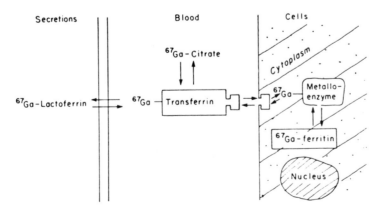

Fig. 13–1. A proposed mechanism for ^{67}Ga uptake into tumor cells. (From Larson, SM: Mechanisms of localization of gallium-67 in tumors. Semin Nucl Med 8:193–204, July 1978, by permission.)

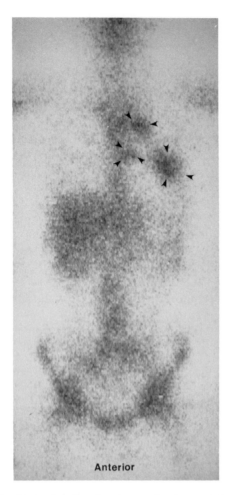

Fig. 13–2. Anterior chest image of patient with lymphoma. Image obtained 48 hours after injection of 5 mC: ^{67}Ga-citrate shows increased uptake in the left lung and mediastinal node areas *(arrows)*.

There are no known contraindications to the use of ^{67}Ga-citrate.

13.3 OTHER TUMOR-SEEKING RADIOPHARMACEUTICALS-RADIOLABELED ANTIBODIES

Antibodies, or immunoglobulins (Ig) (Fig. 13–3), are produced by the activity of the B lymphocytes and possess regions that recognize and bind onto particular sites on antigenic substances. This immunologic response, whenever antibody-antigen binding occurs, usually results in the destruction or elimination of the antigen.

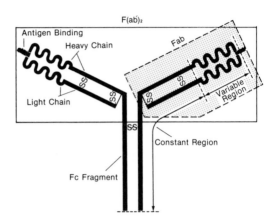

Fig. 13–3. Basic structure of antibody (immunoglobulin, [Ig]) and its various immunologic components. IgG molecules consist of two heavy and two light protein chains held together by disulfide bonds.

An antigen may have one or more sites, each of which can cause the formation of an immunoglobulin that is specific for that antigenic determinant. For this reason, whenever an antigenic challenge occurs, the result is the production of a variety of antibodies.

Originally in nuclear medicine, antibodies employed for tumor detection were derived from an animal (usually a mouse or rabbit) that had been immunized with an antigenic substance. These antibodies are polyspecific because they react against a wide variety of antigenic binding sites (not always limited to tumor). In nuclear medicine, the use of these radiolabeled antibodies obtained from polyclonal sources usually required some type of image enhancement technique (i.e., computer-assisted blood pool subtraction) in order to obtain adequate images.

Highly specific antibodies can be developed by extracting individual lymphocytes and cloning them in tissue culture, with each clone having the potential to develop a single antibody species (a *monoclonal* antibody). Nobel laureates Kohler and Milstein recognized that myeloma cells, which are cancer cells that produce large amounts of identical but nonspecific immunoglobulins, might be altered by recombinant ge-

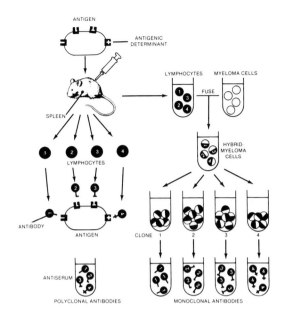

Fig. 13–4. Injection of antigen into mouse or other higher animal elicits heterogeneous antibody response due to stimulation of several B lymphocytes by various determinants on antigen, resulting in polyclonal antibodies in serum (left). If sensitized lymphocytes are removed from spleen of immunized animal and induced to fuse with myeloma cells, individual hybrid cells can be cloned, each producing monoclonal antibodies to single antigenic determinant (right). (From Keenan, AM, Harbert, JC, Larson, SM: Monoclonal antibodies in nuclear medicine. J Nucl Med 26:531–537, 1985, with permission.)

netics and could be used to construct clones that secrete these immunoglobulin products (Fig. 13–4).

Monoclonal cell lines are produced by fusing lymphocytes from the spleen of an immunized mouse with mouse myeloma cells, thus forming clones of hybrid cell lines, called hybridomas. These cells are ordinarily fused in polyethylene glycol media (Fig. 13–5) and result in clones that have the antibody characteristics of the lymphocyte and the longevity of the myeloma cells. Additionally, pure hybridoma cell lines are grown in hypoxanthine-aminopterin-thymidine (HAT) media since it supports neither the unfused lymphocytes nor the myeloma cells. Once hybridomas are produced, further assessment of antibody activity and selective cloning can occur.

Clinical testing of selected radiolabeled monoclonal antibodies directed against tumor antigens is under way using antibodies against oncofetal antigens (alphafetoprotein), placental antigens (human chorionic gonadotrophin, placental alkaline phosphatase), and other tissue or organ-associated antigens including carcinoembryonic antigen (CEA) and an antimelanoma antibody called "p97."

Recently, clinical investigators have sought to hasten tumor uptake and decrease levels of nontumor antibody in blood by preparing small fragments of monoclonal antibodies (Fig. 13–6). These small antibody fragments, called Fab and F(ab')$_2$, possess antigenic specificity without other Ig properties.

13.4 LYMPHOSCINTIGRAPHY

Lymphoscintigraphy was initially evaluated as a potential method for radiation therapy of metastatic spread of breast cancer to mammary lymphatics and used β^- emitting radiopharmaceuticals such as Au-198 colloid. Although the therapeutic goal was not attained, lymphoscintigraphy has proven useful for the visualization and assessment of lymph node groups in patients with rectal and prostate carcinoma, gynecologic tumors, melanoma, and lower extremity edema secondary to lymphatic obstruction. Lymphoscintigraphy is particularly beneficial in the management of breast cancer; approximately 25% of all patients with operable breast cancer will have internal mammary node metastases.

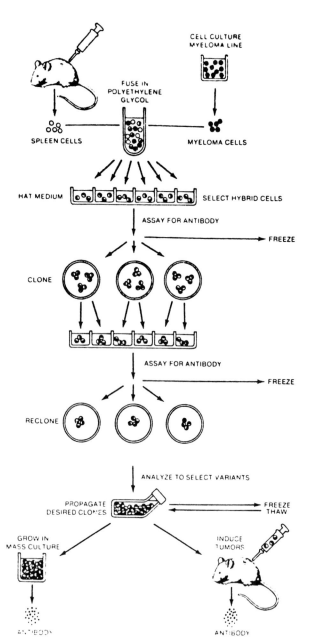

Fig. 13–5. Fusion of antigen-stimulated spleen cells with myeloma cells in polyethylene glycol results in hybrid cells that can be cloned in HAT medium. Those clones that generate immunoglobulin are further propagated, and those producing antibodies to desired antigen are selected to find variant that produces antibody with desired specificity and binding properties. Hybridomas can be maintained in mass culture or mouse ascites, and clones at any stage of development can be frozen for later use. (From Keenan, AM, Harbert, JC, Larson, SM: Monoclonal antibodies in nuclear medicine. J Nucl Med 26:531–537, 1985, with permission.)

Principle

Selected radiocolloids, when administered interstitially, will be actively and passively transported from the injection site to lymph nodes by lymph flow and macrophages. The lymph-carrying radiocolloid enters a node through afferent subcapsular lymphatics (Fig. 13–7), and the radiopharmaceutical is trapped within the sinusoids or actively phagocytized by reticuloendothelial cells in the lymph node.

Indications

The uses of lymphoscintigraphy are shown in Table 13–5. With breast carci-

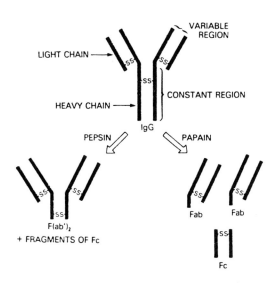

Fig. 13–6. Variable regions of IgG bind specific antigenic sites while the constant region interacts with the host immune system. Enzymatic digestion of disulfide bonds with pepsin removes part of constant region to produce an F(ab')₂ fragment, whereas papain splits molecule into Fc fragment and two Fab fragments. (From Keenan, AM, Harbert, JC, Larson, SM: Monoclonal antibodies in nuclear medicine. J Nucl Med 26:531–537, 1985, with permission.)

nomas, internal mammary node lymphoscintigraphy allows visualization and comparison of the right and left internal mammary chains (Fig. 13–8) and provides a means of localizing lymphatic nodal groups for greater accuracy in radiation therapy treatment planning. Determining the location of the internal mammary nodes is important because standard mediastinal radiation ports and tangential chest wall ports do not allow for variability in the location of nodes. In other words, unless the nodes are visualized, they may lie outside the radiation treatment port, resulting in inadequate therapy.

Radiopharmaceutical Data

The radiocolloid of choice for lymphoscintigraphy is ⁹⁹ᵐTc-antimony sulfide colloid (⁹⁹ᵐTc-SbSC). This radiopharmaceutical is a homogeneous, monodispersion colloid that has uniformly smaller particle size (ranging from 3 to 30 nm) than ⁹⁹ᵐTc-sulfur colloid. Additionally, lymphatic uptake of ⁹⁹ᵐTc-antimony sulfide colloid has been shown to be more efficient when compared to other colloids.

Method

As previously mentioned, ⁹⁹ᵐTc-SbSC is administered interstitially (Fig. 13–9) usually in very high specific activity. A tuberculin syringe with a 1.5-in 22-G needle is usually preferred, and a small volume of air is usually placed behind the radiopharmaceutical to ensure the delivery of the entire amount of the radiocolloid. The radiopharmaceutical volume should be as small as possible and should not exceed 0.3 ml.

In patients with breast carcinoma, the radiopharmaceutical is initially injected at the subcostal site on the same side as or ipsilateral to the breast cancer. Three hours later an anterior chest image is obtained, after which an injection is made to the contralateral injection site. Images are again obtained three hours later.

Special Considerations/Patient Preparation

Proper administration of ⁹⁹ᵐTc-SbSC is critical for obtaining diagnostically useful images. If the radiopharmaceutical is administered too deeply (i.e., past the posterior rectus sheath and into the peritoneal cavity), intraperitoneal radioactivity will be noted and visualization of the parasternal lymphatics may be variable. If the radiopharmaceutical is administered superficially, the axillary nodes may be demonstrated or there may be inconsistent visualization of the internal mammary nodes.

13.5 STUDIES OF HEMATOLOGIC FUNCTION

Several studies of hematologic function can be performed using radiopharmaceut-

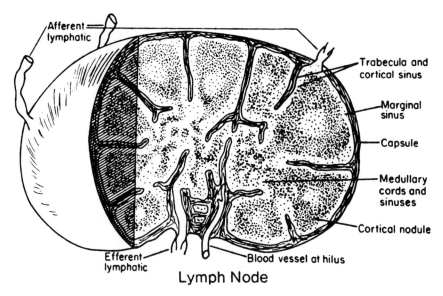

Lymph Node

Fig. 13–7. Cross sectional anatomy of a lymph node. (From Burchiel, SW, Rhodes, BA: Tumor Imaging: The Radioimmunochemical Detection of Cancer. New York, Masson Publishing, 1982.)

Table 13–5. Clinical uses of lymphoscintigraphy.

1. Indicating anatomic direction of lymph drainage
2. Making preoperative estimate of metastases
3. Selecting appropriate therapy
4. Defining necessary radiation therapy portals

icals. These include (1) ferrokinetics, (2) red blood cell mass, (3) red blood cell survival, (4) red blood cell sequestration, (5) radio-labeling of blood cell components (platelets, leukocytes, and fibrinogen), and (6) imaging of hematopoietic (bone marrow) tissues.

13.6 FERROKINETICS

Radioisotopes of iron (primarily Fe-59) can be used to determine the amount of iron absorbed, transported, stored, utilized, and excreted. The most commonly employed tests of ferrokinetics are: iron clearance from the plasma, plasma iron turnover, the utilization of iron in new red blood cells (RBCs), and iron turnover in the liver, spleen, and bone marrow.

The Internal Mammary Nodes

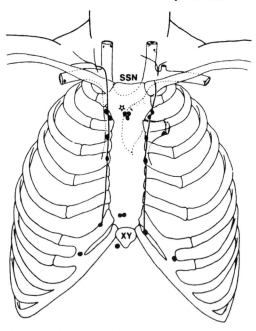

Fig. 13–8. Parasternal location of right and left internal mammary nodes, xiphisternal nodes, and superior mediastinum nodal crossover. (From Burchiel, SW, Rhodes, BA: Tumor Imaging: The Radioimmunochemical Detection of Cancer. New York, Masson Publishing, 1982.)

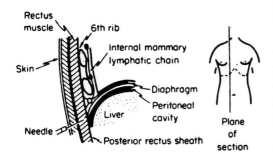

Fig. 13–9. Cross table and anterior views of injection technique for ^{99m}Tc-antimony sulfide colloid (^{99m}TcSbSC) for lymphoscintigraphy of the internal mammary nodes. (From Burchiel, SW, Rhodes, BA: Tumor Imaging. The Radioimmunochemical Detection of Cancer. New York, Masson Publishing, 1982.)

Principle

Because iron is incorporated into hemoglobin during RBC production, the use of radioactive iron provides insight into the effectiveness of erythropoiesis and sites at which it occurs. Since the disappearance of radioiron from the plasma is normally due to uptake by the bone marrow during hemoglobin synthesis, the use of radioiron provides diagnostic information in patients with anemias.

Indications

Failure of radioiron to disappear from the plasma (the normal half-life in serum is 1 to 2 hours) occurs in conditions such as aplastic anemia, hemochromatosis, myelofibrosis, and leukemia that inhibit normal iron uptake by the bone marrow. Disappearance of iron at a greater than normal rate occurs in anemias in which iron uptake is not impaired, such as in iron deficiency, anemia, and infection. Normal serum iron values and those in various disease states are shown in Figure 13–10.

Early uptake of iron by the liver and spleen at a greater than normal rate is an indication of red blood cell formation outside the marrow (extramedullary erythropoietic activity), while uptake by only the spleen at a later time may indicate sequestration of red blood cells.

Radiopharmaceutical Data

Of the available radioisotopes of iron, Fe-59 is usually preferred, although its high-energy gamma rays (1.095 and 1.29 MeV) do not permit acceptable spatial resolution

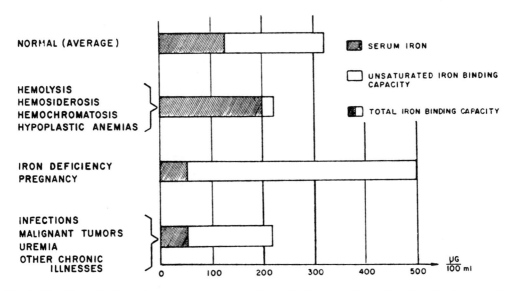

Fig. 13–10. Normal values of serum iron, unsaturated iron binding capacity, and total iron binding capacity, and values in various disease states. (From Harbert, JC, Rocha, AFG (eds.): Textbook of Nuclear Medicine: Clinical Applications. Philadelphia, Lea & Febiger, 1979.)

Table 13–6. Steps involved in the tagging of red blood cells with ^{51}Cr-sodium chromate (^{51}Cr-Na$_2$-CrO$_4$).

1. Incubate whole blood with ^{51}Cr-Na$_2$CrO$_4$ (50–300 μCi).
2. Stop cell labeling by adding ascorbic acid.
3. Wash noncellular Cr-51 from preparation.
4. Reinject ^{51}Cr-labeled red blood cells.

with existing imaging systems. Fe-59 is easily measured in blood samples and can be detected in vivo by external probes over localization sites. Since Fe-55 emits only low-energy x rays, it is useless for external detection and difficult to measure in blood samples. Fe-52, a positron emitter, is not suitable for ferrokinetic studies because its short physical half-life (8.5 hours) prohibits studies of iron metabolism being carried out over the required 8 to 10 days.

Methods

Usually, 5 to 10 μCi of Fe-59 as ferrous citrate is administered by intravenous injection. The radioiron should be bound initially to transferrin either by prior incubation with plasma or by slow injection.

To determine the initial clearance rate of iron from plasma, blood samples are drawn at intervals, starting at about 5 minutes and extending over a period of 1 to 2 hours.

The rate of incorporation of radioactive iron into circulating RBCs is determined by calculating the percentage of injected iron reappearing in the blood.

At the time the study is begun, a standard of the Fe-59 is prepared. The amount of Fe-59 incorporated into RBCs is determined by comparing the counting rate of a sample of the patient's blood (multiplied by the patient's RBC volume) to a standard to represent the activity injected.

13.7 ^{51}Cr-RED BLOOD CELL MASS

When incubated with blood, Cr-51 will "tag" red blood cells and remain within the red cell as long as the cell is viable. Only

the hexavalent state of Cr-51 (Na$_2$CrO$_4$) binds red blood cells. In the in vitro labeling process, a reducing agent, such as ascorbic acid, is added to the cells to reduce Cr-51 (VI) to Cr-51(III) to stop the cell tagging. Nontagged Cr-51 can be removed by cell washing (Table 13–6). After reinjection, Cr-51 from the red blood cells will not reenter other erythrocytes, apparently because the previously bound Cr-51 has been chemically altered. The 27.8-day physical half-life of Cr-51 allows for long-term study of red blood cell kinetics, and its principal photon emission (300 KeV) can be readily detected. By tagging a known volume of the patient's red blood cells with Cr-51, reinjecting the cells, and measuring the activity in a second volume of blood (after allowing sufficient time for mixing), the blood volume and the red cell volume (mass) can be calculated (Table 13–7).

$$\text{RBC volume} = \frac{\text{activity injected} \ (0.92)^* \times \text{hematocrit}}{\text{activity/ml of whole blood}}$$

$$\text{Blood volume} = \frac{\text{activity injected}}{\text{activity/ml of whole blood}}$$

Determination of red cell volume is useful in the differential diagnosis of polycythemia and in following the response to therapy of patients with polycythemia.

13.8 RED BLOOD CELL SURVIVAL

The rate of disappearance of red blood cells from the circulation can also be studied with Cr-51–labeled erythrocytes. Cr-51 labeling must be carefully performed to avoid damaging the red cells and altering their normal life span. Using serial blood samples drawn at 3 to 5-day intervals over 10 to 30 days, a measure of the rate of disappearance of red blood cells (which relates to life span) can be obtained. A sample taken at 24 hours after reinjection of Cr-51–labeled red cells is designated the

---

*Correction factor for plasma trapped with RBCs in hematocrit determination.

Table 13–7. Normal blood volume compartment values (ml/kg).

	Males	Females
Total blood volume	55–80	50–75
Red cell volume[a]	25–35	20–30
Plasma volume[b]	30–45	30–45

[a]95% confidence limits
[b]Because of the many variables that may influence plasma volume in normals, it is not possible to place confidence limits on these values.
From: Rocha, AFG, Harbert, JC (eds.): Textbook on Nuclear Medicine: Clinical Applications. Philadelphia, Lea & Febiger, 1979, p. 403.

100% value, and all other samples are counted and compared to this standard.

Red blood cell survival studies are helpful in evaluating patients with anemia of unknown cause when a hemolytic process is suspected.

13.9 RED BLOOD CELL SEQUESTRATION

Cr-51 tagged red blood cells can also be used to study cell sequestration. The major site for the removal of dying red cells is the spleen, although Cr-51 released from dying cells will also accumulate in the liver. Because of the larger mass of the liver (compared to the spleen), external detection over the liver and spleen normally yields approximately equal ratios. In hypersplenism, however, the spleen destroys red cells at an abnormally high rate, causing a much higher spleen/liver ratio.

13.10 RADIOLABELING OF OTHER BLOOD CELL COMPONENTS

Platelets. Platelets can be separated from whole blood by differential centrifugation and labeled with Cr-51 to study platelet survival. Platelet survival determined from the blood radioactivity disappearance curve is useful in the evaluation of patients with thrombocytopenia. Sites of platelet sequestration can also be determined.

Platelets can also be labeled with In-111 for external imaging to detect sites of platelet aggregation (clots, etc.) in patients with thrombophlebitis. The procedure for la-

beling platelets with In-111 is detailed in Chapter 8.

Leukocytes. Autologous white blood cells (leukocytes) labeled with ^{111}In-oxine are useful for abscess localization, particularly when the abdomen is the suspected site of the abscess (Ga-67 citrate, the primary abscess-localizing radiopharmaceutical, is normally excreted by the gut). The preparation and use of In-111–labeled leukocytes are discussed in Chapter 8.

Fibrinogen. Radioiodinated fibrinogen (like endogenous fibrinogen) is incorporated into the actively forming thrombus and can be used for clot localization. Depending upon the radiolabel employed, the location of the thrombus can be detected either by hand-held probe-type detectors (using ^{125}I-labeled fibrinogen) or by scintillation imaging (using ^{131}I-labeled fibrinogen).

The test has two drawbacks: (1) usefulness is limited postoperatively because of high levels of fibrinogen normally found in areas of relative hyperemia, and (2) in vivo detection of ^{125}I-labeled fibrinogen is restricted to the use of hand-held probes, and accurate detection of clot formation with hand-held probes is difficult and requires a relatively high degree of experience by the clinician performing the procedure.

13.11 IMAGING OF HEMATOPOIETIC (BONE MARROW) TISSUES

The bone marrow contains hematopoietic cells, which are essential for blood cell formation and the sustaining of life.

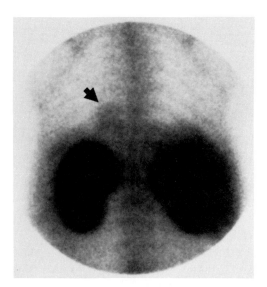

Fig. 13–11. Bone marrow study performed with ^{111}In-chloride demonstrating the site of extramedullary hematopoiesis *(arrow)*.

The bone marrow also contains a fraction of the cells of the reticuloendothelial (RE) system, which can, under certain pathologic conditions, play a significant role in normal body defense mechanisms. The functional assessment of bone marrow is important for diagnostic, prognostic, and therapeutic purposes.

Principles and Radiopharmaceutical Data

Hematopoietic Function. Although radioisotopes of iron are the logical agents for assessment of hemopoietic function, the readily available radioisotopes of iron have either long physical half-lives, poor decay schemes, or principal photon energies unsuitable for scintillation imaging.

Ionic indium (In^{+3}), when injected intravenously, binds to serum transferrin and distributes in a manner analogous to iron. The localization of indium in bone marrow has been shown to follow that of iron, particularly in the early phases of iron uptake by bone marrow (Fig. 13–11). In-111 (as the chloride salt) is the most commonly employed radioisotope of indium for bone

marrow studies although a significant amount of this radiopharmaceutical is also taken up by the liver. For bone marrow imaging 1 to 3 mCi of ^{111}In-chloride is given intravenously and images are obtained 18 to 24 hours later.

Reticuloendothelial (RE) Bone Marrow Imaging. Intravenously administered radioactive colloids are also phagocytized by the RE cells of the bone marrow. Although less than 10% of the RE mass resides in bone marrow, uptake of radioactive colloid is sufficient for satisfactory visualization.

Several factors influence the biological distribution of colloids. Compared to reticuloendothelial cells of the liver and spleen, the RE cells of the bone marrow selectively phagocytize relatively smaller colloid particles (i.e., those less than 100 to 200 mμ in diameter). Severe liver disease such as cirrhosis causes shifts in colloid distribution (with greater uptake in bone marrow). For bone marrow imaging, between 10 and 12 mCi of ^{99m}Tc-sulfur colloid is intravenously administered, and images are obtained approximately 30 minutes later.

While bone marrow imaging is not a commonly employed procedure, it is useful for localizing and defining the extent of hematologic diseases such as leukemia, anemia, and lymphoma. It can also be used to distinguish areas of bone marrow infarction in sickle cell anemia and is helpful in localizing sites for bone marrow biopsy.

REFERENCES

1. Bragg, DG, Hendee, WR: Tumor Imaging: Current State of the Art and Recommendations for Future Research. East Norwalk, CT, Appleton-Century-Crofts, 1982.
2. Blahd, WH (ed.): Nuclear Medicine (2nd ed). New York, McGraw-Hill, 1971, pp. 821.
3. Burchiel, SW, Rhodes, BA: Tumor Imaging: The Radioimmunochemical Detection of Cancer. New York, Masson Publishing, 1982.
4. Eges, G: Lymphoscintigraphy-techniques and applications in the management of breast cancer. Semin Nucl Med 13:26–34, 1983.
5. Hayes, RC: The medical use of gallium radionuclides: A brief history with some comments. Semin Nucl Med 8:183–192, July 1978.
6. Jeffcoat, MK, McNeil, BJ, Davis, MA: Indium and

iron as tracers for erythroid precursors. J Nucl Med 19:496–500, 1978.

7. Keenan, AM, Harbert, JC, Larson, SM: Monoclonal antibodies in nuclear medicine. J Nucl Med 26:531–537, 1985.

8. Larson, SM: Mechanisms of localization of gallium-67 in tumor. Semin Nucl Med 8:193–204, July 1978.

9. Packer, S: Tumor detection with radiopharmaceuticals. Semin Nucl Med 14:21–30, 1984.

10. Staab, EV, McCartney, WH: Role of gallium-67 in inflammatory disease. Semin Nucl Med 8:219–234, July 1978.

11. Thakur, ML, Gottschalk, A (eds.): Indium-111 labeled neutrophils, platelets and lymphocytes. New York, Trivirum Publishing Co., 1980, pp. 213.

14

Radiopharmaceuticals for Skeletal and Renal Imaging

14.1 SKELETAL IMAGING

Destructive bone lesions are produced by a variety of pathologic conditions, including neoplastic disease, metabolic disorders, and infections. Unfortunately, the early detection of bone lesions by routine x rays is difficult since bone demineralization changes of 30 to 50% must occur before density changes can be distinguished on x ray films. This is particularly true for lesions less than 2 cm.

Nuclear medicine bone imaging is considerably more sensitive than conventional x rays for identifying the presence and extent of bone lesions because bone-seeking radiopharmaceuticals usually localize in skeletal lesions very early in the pathologic process. In fact, nuclear medicine techniques often show such abnormalities months before they are visible on routine x ray films.

Principle

Bone-seeking radiopharmaceuticals localize by behaving similarly to normal bone constituents or as a result of affinity for bone. In disease and trauma, localized increased bone metabolic activity and blood flow account for the generally greater concentration (or uptake) of these agents in lesions relative to normal bone (although occasionally entirely destructive skeletal lesions often fail to show any accumulation of bone-seeking radiopharmaceuticals).

Table 14–1. Indications for skeletal imaging.

1.	To screen preoperative patients with malignancies known to metastasize early to bone (e.g., breast, lung, and prostate).
2.	To detect metastatic bone lesions prior to their appearance on x-rays.
3.	To determine the extent of known primary and metastatic lesions.
4.	To localize lesions prior to bone biopsies.
5.	To assist in the planning of radiotherapy portals.
6.	To assess benefit of therapy on bone cancer.
7.	To diagnose osteomyelitis and Paget's disease.
8.	To diagnose stress fractures.

Indications

The highly sensitive nature of skeletal imaging for alterations in bone metabolism makes this technique useful in a variety of pathologic situations (Table 14–1).

Radiopharmaceutical Data

In the early days of nuclear medicine, skeletal imaging was performed using agents such as radiostrontium (Sr-85 and Sr-87m nitrate) and F-18 sodium fluoride. These agents were replaced during the early 1970s when Tc-99m–labeled bone-seeking radiopharmaceuticals became available for skeletal imaging. The development of these agents made it possible to extend the highly desirable imaging properties of Tc-99m to skeletal imaging. Since the introduction of the original Tc-99m–labeled polyphosphate by Subramanian, other Tc-99m radiopharmaceuticals

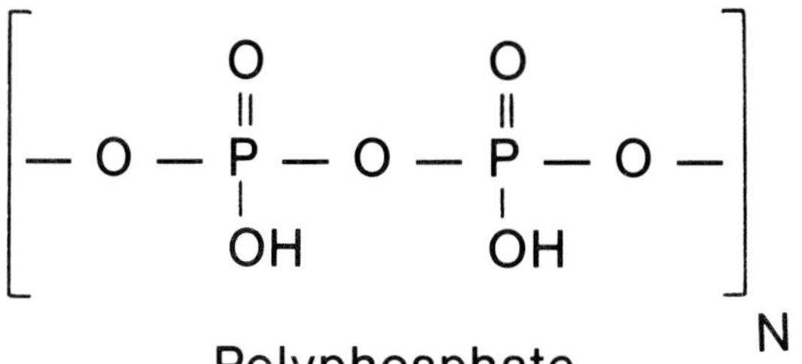

$$\left[-O - \overset{\overset{\displaystyle O}{\|}}{\underset{\underset{\displaystyle OH}{|}}{P}} - O - \overset{\overset{\displaystyle O}{\|}}{\underset{\underset{\displaystyle OH}{|}}{P}} - O - \right]_N$$

Polyphosphate

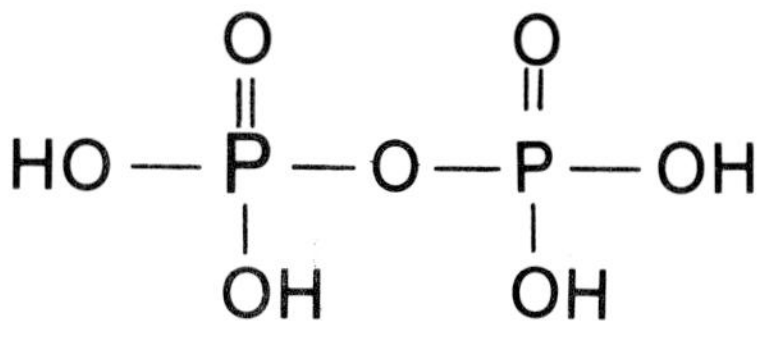

$$HO - \overset{\overset{\displaystyle O}{\|}}{\underset{\underset{\displaystyle OH}{|}}{P}} - O - \overset{\overset{\displaystyle O}{\|}}{\underset{\underset{\displaystyle OH}{|}}{P}} - OH$$

Pyrophosphate

$$HO - \overset{\overset{\displaystyle O}{\|}}{\underset{\underset{\displaystyle OH}{|}}{P}} - \overset{\overset{\displaystyle R_1}{|}}{\underset{\underset{\displaystyle R_2}{|}}{C}} - \overset{\overset{\displaystyle O}{\|}}{\underset{\underset{\displaystyle OH}{|}}{P}} - OH$$

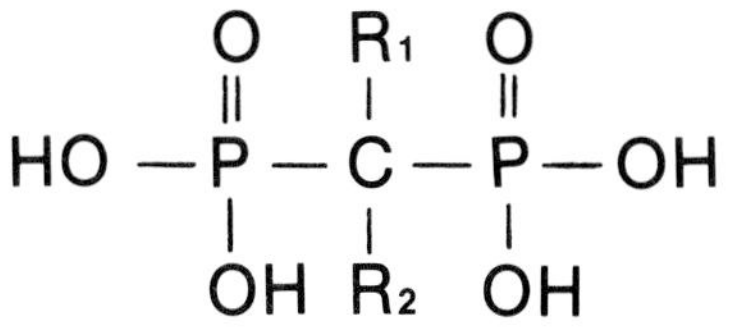

Basic Diphosphonate Structure

Diphosphonate Derivatives	R_1	R_2
Methylene diphosphonate (MDP, also known as medronate)	–H	–H
Hydroxymethylene diphosphonate (HMDP or HDP, also known as oxidronate)	–OH	–H

Fig. 14–1. Chemical configuration of bone-seeking Tc-99m radiopharmaceuticals.

have been developed that have improved biodistribution properties (Fig. 14–1). Unlike the early Tc-99m polyphosphate agent, the Tc-99m–labeled diphosphonates are resistant to in vivo degradation and have higher uptake in bone and more rapid blood clearance. ^{99m}Tc-medronate (MDP) and ^{99m}Tc-oxidronate (HMDP or HDP) are currently the agents of choice for bone imaging. While these agents share the central diphosphonate configuration, slight differences in their chemical structure affect rates of blood clearance and bone uptake. The more rapid blood clearance of ^{99m}Tc-HMDP (Fig. 14–2) usually results in bone images of higher quality than those images obtained with ^{99m}Tc-MDP. It appears, however, that no significant differences exist between the ability of either radiopharmaceutical to detect skeletal metastases.

The precise mechanism of bone localization for the Tc-99m–labeled bone-seekers is not fully understood, although it is generally accepted that localization occurs by chemiadsorption of these agents onto the surface of active hydroxyapatite bone crystal. In diseases affecting bone or in bone trauma, localized increased uptake of the radiopharmaceutical occurs as a result of the relatively greater bone metabolic activity in the involved area (Fig. 14–3). Additionally, hyperemia is an important secondary factor accounting for increased availability of the agent at the bone repair site.

Approximately 50% of an injected dose of either ^{99m}Tc-MDP or ^{99m}Tc-HMDP localizes in bone within 3 to 4 hours after intravenous administration, and the remaining 50% is excreted in the urine over 24 hours. About 10% of the injected dose remains in blood at 1 hour after injection, 5% at 2 hours, and less than 1% at 24 hours. With either radiopharmaceutical, the critical organ is the bladder wall, which receives approximately 3 rads from a dose of 20 mCi.

Method

Approximately 15 to 20 mCi of either ^{99m}Tc-MDP or ^{99m}Tc-HMDP is given intra-

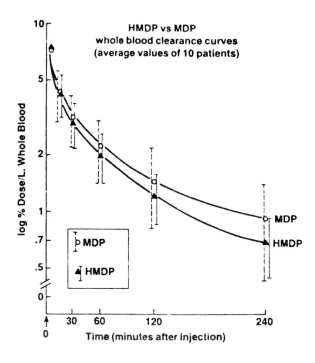

HMDP vs MDP
whole blood clearance curves
(average values of 10 patients)

log % Dose/L. Whole Blood

MDP

HMDP

○ MDP

▲ HMDP

Time (minutes after injection)

Fig. 14–2. Comparative whole blood clearance of Tc-99m HMDP and MDP. (From Littlefield, JL, Rudd, TG: Tc-99m hydroxymethylene diphosphonate and Tc-99m methylene diphosphonate: biological and clinical comparison: concise communication. J Nucl Med 24:463–466, 1983, with permission.)

A   B

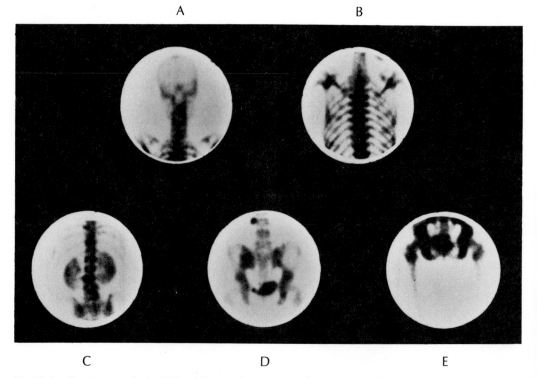

C   D   E

Fig. 14–3. Bone images obtained 2 hrs following intravenous administration of 20 mCi ⁹⁹ᵐTc-MDP. The images show uptake of the radiopharmaceutical in bone with regions of increased pathology: A. Normal, B. Diffuse disease in ribs, C. Multiple lesions in vertebrae, D. Lesions in spine and right pelvis, and E. abnormal right hip joint.

venously, and scintillation images are obtained 2 to 3 hours later. Patients should be encouraged to void immediately prior to imaging since the appearance of the radiopharmaceutical in the urine and bladder could obscure visualization of pelvic bone lesions. (Occasionally, information pertaining to renal function disorders, such as urinary obstruction or kidney blood flow abnormalities, is obtained during bone imaging because of the significant activities normally excreted by the kidneys.)

Special Considerations/Patient Preparation

No special patient preparation is required except for encouraging patients to void immediately before imaging. Metallic objects (jewelry, belt-buckles, etc.) and some prosthetic devices may attenuate photons and thus mimic the appearance of necrotic "photon-deficient" lesions. These materials should be removed prior to imaging.

14.2   RADIOPHARMACEUTICALS USED FOR KIDNEY IMAGING AND STUDIES OF RENAL FUNCTION

Early nuclear medicine studies of renal function were performed with contrast agents that had been made radioactive by radioiodination, usually with I-131. These radiopharmaceuticals were unsatisfactory for renal studies because excretion of these agents often was not limited to the kidneys. Since those early days, radiopharmaceuticals have been developed that are excreted predominantly by the kidneys. Radioactive substances excreted either by glomerular filtration or tubular secretion are useful in evaluating renal function, while radiopharmaceuticals either slowly excreted or bound within the renal cortex are useful for imaging renal anatomy.

Since renal handling mechanisms largely determine clinical usefulness, the discussion of these agents will be based upon the specific renal excretion mechanism. Radiopharmaceuticals excreted by glomerular filtration will be presented first.

14.3   AGENTS EXCRETED PREDOMINANTLY BY GLOMERULAR FILTRATION

- ^{99m}Tc-DTPA (pentetate, or diethylenetriamine pentaacetic acid)
- ^{99m}Tc-sodium pertechnetate

Indications

Radiopharmaceuticals excreted by glomerular filtration are useful in analyzing renal blood flow, determining glomerular filtration rate, and visualizing the urinary collection system.

Radiopharmaceutical Data

^{99m}Tc-DTPA is a "pure" glomerular agent; that is, its only mode of renal excretion is glomerular filtration. Additionally, there is no appreciable reabsorption of ^{99m}Tc-DTPA in the renal tubules. The concentration of ^{99m}Tc-DTPA in the kidneys reaches a peak approximately 3 to 4 minutes after intravenous injection. At 2 hours after injection, almost 50% of the dose is excreted in the urine, and nearly 95% by 24 hours. Very little ^{99m}Tc-DTPA is retained in the kidney (3 to 4% at 1 hour and only 1% at 24 hours).

^{99m}Tc-sodium pertechnetate can be used for studying renal blood flow since it also is cleared by glomerular filtration. Pertechnetate, however, is extensively bound to serum protein ($\approx$85%) and has a very slow rate of renal clearance, with approximately 85% of filtered ^{99m}Tc-sodium pertechnetate reabsorbed in the renal tubules. For these reasons, ^{99m}Tc-sodium pertechnetate is generally useful only for determining the adequacy of renal blood flow (the single mode of excretion of ^{99m}Tc-DTPA usually

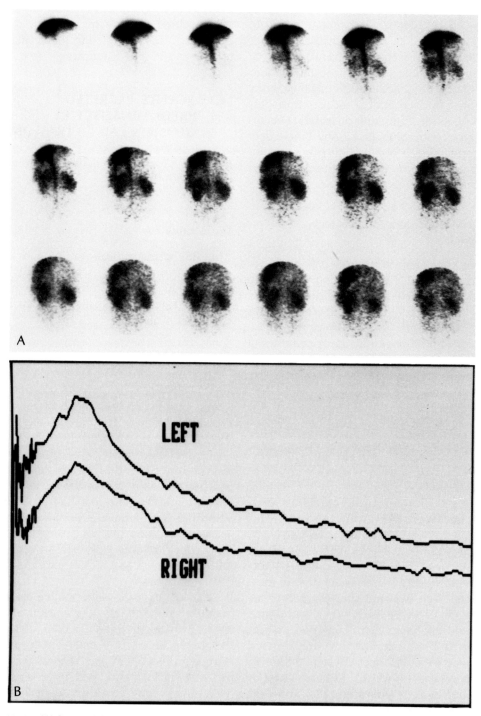

Fig. 14–4. (A) Series of dynamic images obtained upon injection of ^{99m}Tc-DTPA at 5-second intervals. Kidneys show apparent uniform perfusion and clearance of this radiopharmaceutical. (B) Computer-derived tracings over kidneys obtained after injection of ^{99m}Tc-DTPA.

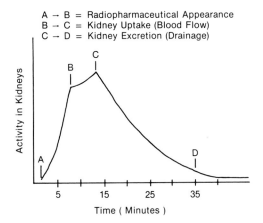

A → B = Radiopharmaceutical Appearance
B → C = Kidney Uptake (Blood Flow)
C → D = Kidney Excretion (Drainage)

Fig. 14–5. A schematic representation of a computer-derived renogram in a patient with normal renal function. The three segments of radiopharmaceutical clearance (radiopharmaceutical appearance, blood flow, and drainage) are shown.

makes this agent preferable for studies seeking to quantify renal blood flow).

Method

Rapid sequence images are obtained immediately after the intravenous administration of 15 mCi of ^{99m}Tc-DTPA (usually at 5- to 10-second intervals) for 1 to 2 minutes, with subsequent images taken at 5-minute intervals for approximately 30 minutes (Fig. 14–4).

Computer-assisted evaluation of radiopharmaceutical uptake and clearance by the kidneys is a useful technique in the diagnosis of renal function. This method, which produces a *renogram*, provides diagnostic information relating to renal problems affecting renal function (or blood supply) and those causing urinary tract obstruction.

A schematic representation of a normal renogram is shown in Figure 14–5. The three segments of radiopharmaceutical uptake and clearance by the kidneys demonstrate various components of renal function.

The estimated radiation dose for ^{99m}Tc-DTPA to the critical organ, the bladder, is

3.5 rads per 15 mCi, while the kidneys receive approximately 1.2 rads.

Special Considerations/Patient Preparation

The patient's state of hydration influences the renal excretion of radiopharmaceuticals and the shape of the computer-derived renogram curve. In dehydrated patients, for example, the time required to reach peak uptake (phase A-B, Fig. 14–5) is prolonged, as are subsequent phases. False differences in rates of radiopharmaceutical excretion may also occur because of increased pooling of highly concentrated urine in slight nonpathologic variations of ureteral outlets.

Because of its rapid renal clearance, ^{99m}Tc-DTPA cannot be adequately imaged with rectilinear imaging devices.

Interventional Agents

The diuretic furosemide (Lasix) can be used as an interventional aid for the renogram to assist in the diagnosis of urinary tract obstructions. This renogram modification primarily involves the administration of the parenteral diuretic after the administration of either Tc-99m pentetate (DTPA) or radioiodinated orthoiodohippuric acid (OIHA). Computer-assisted analysis of kidney, ureter, and bladder activity is derived, and information from these regions of interest is plotted against time as a histogram.

Furosemide increases urine volume and flow rates by inhibiting sodium ion reabsorption from the proximal and distal tubules and from the ascending limb of the loop of Henle. In normal patients or patients with dilated, nonobstructed renal collecting systems, the increased urine volume and flow rates result in a rapid decline or "wash-out" of radioactivity (Fig. 14–6). In the obstructed pattern, however, the kidney time-activity histogram demonstrates a flat response without significant

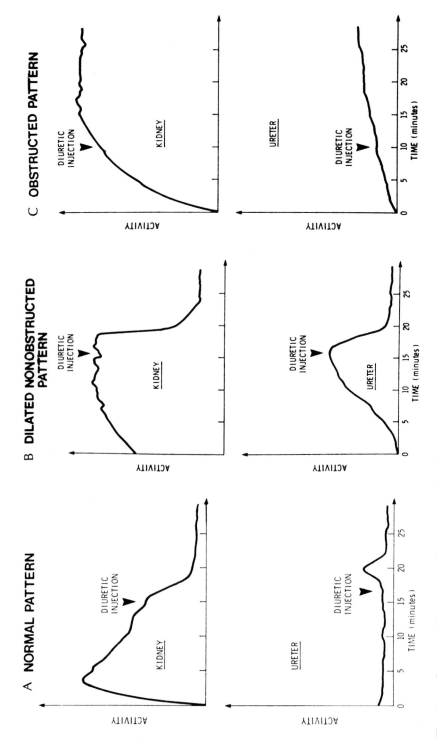

Fig. 14–6. Representative furosemide renograms showing time-activity curve patterns in normal patient (A) and in patients with dilated nonobstruction (B) and obstruction (C) of the urinary collecting systems. (From Thrall, JH, Koff, SA, Keyes, JW, Jr.: Diuretic radionuclide renography and scintgraphy in the differential diagnosis of hydroureteronephrosis. Semin Nucl Med 11(Issue 2):89–104, 1981, with permission.)

Table 14–2.   Comparative radiation dose from ^{123}I- and ^{131}I-OIHA.

	^{123}I-OIHA rads/500 µCi*	^{131}I-OIHA rads/200 µCi*
Bladder wall	0.750	2.4
Thyroid	0.30	8.5
Kidneys	0.03	0.02
Ovaries	0.02	0.01
Testes	0.02	0.01

*Usual adult dose.

and its significantly lower radiation dosimetry (Table 14–2) make it the superior radioiodinated OIHA product. Both of these radiopharmaceuticals are cleared by glomerular filtration (20%) and renal tubular secretion (80%) and have a renal extraction efficiency higher than that of any ^{99m}Tc agent currently employed.

wash-out; the pattern for obstructed ureters is similar (Fig. 14–6). In adults, the usual dose of furosemide is 0.3 to 0.5 mg/kg (maximum dose 40 mg), while children receive 1.0 mg/kg up to a maximum of 20 mg. Generally, furosemide is administered intravenously over a 1- to 2-minute period. Since dehydrated patients should not receive parenteral diuretics, a normal state of hydration is recommended whenever furosemide renography is indicated.

14.4   AGENTS THAT ARE PREDOMINANTLY SECRETED

• ^{131}I-orthoiodohippurate (OIHA, or orthoiodohippuric acid)
• ^{123}I-orthoiodohippurate (OIHA, or orthoiodohippuric acid)

Indications

These radiopharmaceuticals are pharmacologically identical and are useful for the quantitation of effective renal plasma flow (ERPF), a diagnostic indicator of renal tubular function. The primary clinical usefulness of this test lies in demonstrating either total or differential renal function.

Radiopharmaceutical Data

Although ^{131}I-OIHA has been the radiopharmaceutical of choice for evaluation of ERPF, the undesirable decay properties of this beta-emitting radionuclide make it unattractive. Recently, OIHA labeled with I-123 has been made available. The more desirable nuclear properties of ^{123}I-OIHA

Method

Because of the relatively high radiation dose to the bladder and thyroid, adult doses of ^{131}I-OIHA usually do not exceed 200 µCi. The favorable decay properties of I-123 allow adult patients to be administered 500 µCi of ^{123}I-OIHA and occasionally as much as 1.0 mCi. With either radiopharmaceutical, imaging is begun soon after injection, usually at 1- to 2-minute intervals continuing for half an hour. Computer-assisted image processing (Fig. 14–7) is useful in determining comparative renal function.

Special Considerations/Patient Preparation

The patient's state of hydration is an important factor influencing radiopharmaceutical uptake and clearance by the kidneys (see Section 14.3 Special Considerations/Patient Preparation).

In patients receiving ^{131}I-OIHA, pretreatment with either Lugol's solution or saturated potassium iodide is suggested in order to block thyroid uptake of free (unbound) I-131.

14.5   AGENTS USEFUL FOR RENAL CORTEX VISUALIZATION (ARCHITECTURAL IMAGING)

• ^{99m}Tc-DMSA (2,3-dimercaptosuccinic acid, or succimer)
• ^{99m}Tc-gluceptate (formerly glucoheptonate)

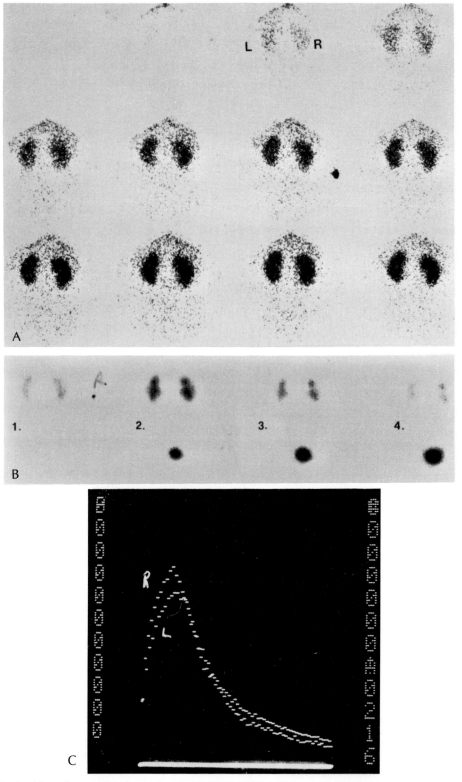

Fig. 14–7. Normal renogram obtained with ¹²³I-OIHA. Image A shows the dynamic appearance of the radiopharmaceutical in kidneys over 10-second intervals. Image B shows radiopharmaceutical uptake and excretion in images taken over 225 seconds each (with dual exposure). Image C is the computer-derived renogram tracing as illustrated in Figure 14–5. (Case provided courtesy of TG Rudd, M.D., Seattle, WA.)

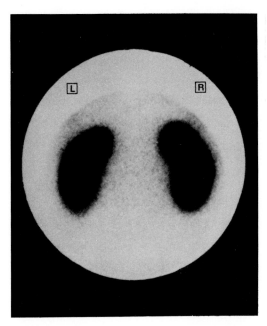

Fig. 14–8. Static-type images of the kidney obtained two hours after injection of ^{99m}Tc-DMSA (succimer).

Indications

Both ^{99m}Tc-DMSA and ^{99m}Tc-gluceptate are useful in determining if renal masses are tumors or "pseudotumors" (e.g., cystic masses) and for obtaining information on kidney size or position.

Radiopharmaceutical Data

^{99m}Tc-DMSA localizes in the renal cortex, reaching a concentration of approximately 25% of the injected dose at 1 hour after injection, increasing to 40% at 6 hours. ^{99m}Tc-gluceptate also localizes in the renal cortex, but the fraction of injected dose (15 to 20%) in the cortex remains relatively constant for 2 to 6 hours after injection (Fig. 14–8).

The renal clearance rate is higher for gluceptate than for ^{99m}Tc-DMSA. At 3 hours, about 50% of the administered dose of gluceptate is recovered in the urine, whereas only 16% of ^{99m}Tc-DMSA is found in the urine over the same time period. As a result, the total body retention of ^{99m}Tc-

DMSA (primarily in the kidneys) is much longer.

Method

Patients are injected intravenously with either 10 to 15 mCi ^{99m}Tc-gluceptate or 3 to 5 mCi ^{99m}Tc-DMSA and are imaged approximately 2 to 4 hours later. With ^{99m}Tc-DMSA, limitations in patient radiation dose (approximately 7 rads to renal cortex with 5 mCi) prohibit the administration of sufficient activity for dynamic imaging of renal blood flow.

Special Considerations/Patient Preparation

^{99m}Tc-gluceptate has demonstrated much greater in vitro stability (higher "tagging efficiency" over longer periods of time) than ^{99m}Tc-DMSA. ^{99m}Tc-DMSA tends to deteriorate rapidly after Tc-99m radiolabeling and must be used within 30 minutes following a 30-minute incubation period from the time of Tc-99m radiolabeling. With either radiopharmaceutical, patients should be in a normal state of hydration.

REFERENCES

Skeletal Imaging

1. Davis, MA, Jones, AG: Comparison of Tc-99m-labeled phosphate and phosphonate agents for skeletal imaging. Semin Nucl Med 6:19–31, 1976.
2. Fogelman, I: Diphosphonate bone scanning agents—current concepts. Eur J Nucl Med 7:506–509, 1982.
3. Jones, AG, Francis, MD, Davis, MA: Bone scanning: radionuclide reactor mechanisms. Semin Nucl Med 6:3–18, 1976.
4. Kirchner, PT (ed.): Nuclear Medicine Review Syllabus. New York, Society of Nuclear Medicine, 1980, pp. 539–586.
5. Koenigsberg, M, Freeman, LM: Radionuclide bone imaging. Curr Probl Diag Radiol 6:1–54, 1976.
6. O'Mara, RE, Charkes, ND: The osseous system. In Clinical Scintillation Imaging. Edited by LM Freeman, PM Johnson. New York, Grune and Stratton, 1975, pp. 537–599.
7. Siegel, BA, Donovan, RL, Alderson, PO, et al.: Skeletal uptake of Tc-99m diphosphonate in re-

lation to local bone blood flow. Radiology *120*:121–123, 1976.

8. Subramanian, G, McAfee, JG: A new complex of Tc-99m for skeletal imaging. Radiology *99*:192–196, 1971.

9. Subramanian, G, McAfee, JG, Thomas, FD, et al.: New diphosphonate compounds for skeletal imaging: comparison with methylene diphosphonate. Radiology *149*:823–828, 1983.

10. Van Duzee, BF, Schaefer, JA, Ball, JD, et al.: Relative lesion detection ability of Tc-99m HMDP and Tc-99m MDP: concise communication. J Nucl Med *25*:166–169, 1984.

Renal

1. Arnold, RW, Subramanian, G, McAfee, JG, et al.: Comparison of Tc-99m complexes for renal imaging. J Nucl Med *16*:357–367, 1975.

2. Chervu, LR, Blaufox, MD: Renal radiopharmaceuticals—an update. Semin Nucl Med *12*:224–245, 1982.

3. Dubovsky, EV, Russell, CD: Quantitation of renal function with glomerular and tubular agents. Semin Nucl Med *12*:330–334, 1982.

4. Freeman, LM, Blaufox, MD (eds.): Radionuclide Studies of the Genitourinary System. New York, Grune and Stratton, 1975.

5. Handmaker, H, Young, B, Lowenstein, J: Clinical experience with Tc-99m-DMSA (dimercaptosuccinic acid): a new renal imaging agent. J Nucl Med *16*:28–32, 1975.

6. Kirchner, PT (ed.): Nuclear Medicine Review Syllabus. New York, Society of Nuclear Medicine, 1980, pp. 323–384.

7. Thrall, JH, Swanson, DP. Diagnostic Interventions in Nuclear Medicine. Chicago, Yearbook Medical Publishers, 1985.

Radiopharmaceuticals for Cardiac Imaging

15.1 CARDIAC IMAGING

Nuclear medicine cardiac studies can be divided into two categories (Table 15–1) based on the clinical information desired. In addition, these two categories—imaging the myocardium and determining quantitative cardiac function—may be further broken into groups based on the specific diagnostic properties of the radiopharmaceuticals used.

15.2 AVID INFARCT IMAGING

Principle

^{99m}Tc-pyrophosphate (^{99m}Tc-PPi) "avid" infarct imaging has been performed since the mid-1970s, when clinicians noted that this bone-seeking radiopharmaceutical concentrated in the chests of patients with previous histories of chest pain. Subsequent investigations revealed that ^{99m}Tc-PPi localization occurred specifically in the injured myocardium.

The uptake mechanism for this radiopharmaceutical in the damaged myocardium is not completely understood. It has been shown, however, that during irreversible tissue injury calcium deposition increases, perhaps resulting in the formation of calcium phosphate complexes much like the hydroxyapatite crystals of bone that act as sites of uptake for Tc-99m bone seekers. It has been postulated that these injury-related substances serve as affinity sites for ^{99m}Tc-PPi in the damaged myocardium. Increased ^{99m}Tc-PPi uptake in the injured myocardium requires that blood flow within the injury site be adequate to provide delivery of the radiopharmaceuticals, yet sufficiently decreased to cause the ischemic injury. The highest ^{99m}Tc-PPi uptake has been shown to occur in the periphery of infarction, where there is 10 to 40% blood flow remaining (decreased but not absent).

Indications

Avid infarct imaging is useful in determining the location of and estimating the

Table 15–1. Classification of nuclear medicine studies of the heart, including the types of radiopharmaceutical localization mechanisms and clinical utility.

Category	Radiopharmaceutical Mechanism Type	Clinical Utility
I. Imaging the myocardium	1. *Avid infarct*—localization of radiopharmaceutical in damaged myocardium only.	Useful in delineating infarction.
	2. *Myocardial perfusion*—localization of agent in viable myocardium only.	Sensitive indicator of perfusion abnormalities.
II. Determining quantitative cardiac function	Computer-assisted acquisition and image processing of *radiopharmaceutical confined to vascular blood pool.*	Useful in evaluating cardiac function (e.g., cardiac ejection fraction).

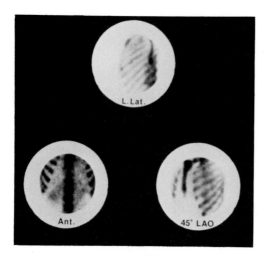

Fig. 15–1. ^{99m}Tc-pyrophosphate (^{99m}Tc-PPi) study performed in a patient with no apparent infarction abnormality.

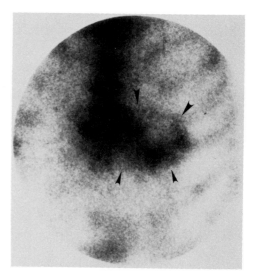

Fig. 15–2. Anterior chest image of patient with a massive myocardial infarction *(arrows)*.

size of acute myocardial infarction and is useful as a screening procedure when electrocardiogram changes are not apparent and serum enzyme levels are not diagnostic. It is also useful in differentiating new and old myocardial infarctions.

Radiopharmaceutical Data

^{99m}Tc-pyrophosphate is the preferred radiopharmaceutical for acute myocardial infarct imaging. Although other ^{99m}Tc-labeled bone seekers have been investigated for infarct imaging and compared to ^{99m}Tc-PPi, none have proven superior for the detection of myocardial infarction.

Methods

In adults, 15 to 20 mCi ^{99m}Tc-PPi is injected intravenously, with scintillation images obtained at least 90 minutes later. Views in anterior, 45° left anterior oblique (LAO), and left lateral positions are routinely obtained (Fig. 15–1). Areas of acute infarction have increased radiopharmaceutical uptake (Fig. 15–2). Myocardial infarction imaging may be performed as early as 18 hours after the acute episode or

within 14 days of the event. Maximum uptake, however, is limited to a shorter time span, usually 2 to 3 days after infarction. Grading of images for the visibility of suspected infarction depends upon the activity within the myocardium (Table 15–2).

Special Considerations/Patient Preparation

No special patient preparation is necessary. It has been reported that trauma, tumor, pericarditis, aneurysm, and amyloidosis may also localize ^{99m}Tc-PPi and result in false positive studies. Diffuse uptake of ^{99m}Tc-PPi may also be the result of cardioversion, and persistent blood pool activity may be responsible for false positive interpretations.

Table 15–2.   Grading of ^{99m}Tc-PPi scintillation images in suspected myocardial infarction.

Grading	Radiopharmaceutical appearance in myocardium
0	No ^{99m}Tc-PPi activity in myocardium.
1+	Minimal activity most likely representing blood pool.
2+	Definite ^{99m}Tc-PPi myocardial uptake.
3+	Myocardial uptake *equal* to bone.
4+	Myocardial uptake *greater* than in bone.

Table 15–3.   Indications for myocardial perfusion imaging.

1. To detect abnormalities in coronary arteries.
2. To locate areas of decreased myocardial blood flow.
3. To evaluate actual physiologic effect of known coronary artery stenosis.
4. To evaluate improvement in blood flow following bypass surgery.
5. To evaluate effects of drug therapy.
6. To identify patients with falsely abnormal EKGs.
7. To evaluate effects of stress on myocardial blood flow.
8. To identify old myocardial infarctions.
9. To identify patients with physiologic angina pectoris.

15.3   MYOCARDIAL PERFUSION IMAGING OF ISCHEMIC HEART DISEASE

Principle

Myocardial imaging can also be performed using radiopharmaceuticals that localize in viable cardiac muscle only. This type of cardiac imaging is called myocardial "perfusion imaging" and should not be confused with avid infarct imaging.

Normally perfused myocardial cells have a high intracellular potassium utilization rate resulting from the high degree of muscle contractility. While other muscle tissues and organs also utilize potassium, the myocardium has the highest concentration of this element per gram of tissue. Although it seems reasonable that this pathway might be useful for myocardial imaging, no radioisotope of potassium exists that has suitable imaging properties. Fortunately Tl-201, an analogue of potassium, is also extracted by the myocardium and has nuclear properties that permit its use for myocardial perfusion studies.

Indications

Tl-201 myocardial perfusion imaging can be used to differentiate the normally perfused myocardium from nonperfused tissues and has several clinical indications (Table 15–3). Since only healthy myocardial tissue extracts Tl-201 from blood, the non-perfused myocardium shows as "cold" areas.

Images obtained immediately following the injection of Tl-201 during exercise stress and at rest are helpful in the diagnosis of exercise-induced ischemia (Table 15–4).

Radiopharmaceutical Data

Tl-201 is administered intravenously as Tl-201 thallous chloride. Following injection, Tl-201 clears rapidly from blood with a half-life of less than two minutes. In the resting state, about 5% of the injected dose localizes in the heart at 15 minutes after injection, with 4% localizing in the kidneys and 12% in the liver. Less than 5% is excreted by the kidneys at 24 hours. The whole-body half-life for Tl-201 thallous chloride is approximately 10 days.

Tl-201 is formed by the decay of accelerator-produced Pb-201 (Fig. 15–3).

The nuclear properties of Tl-201 are shown on Table 15–5. Because they are abundant, the mercury x rays (68–80 KeV) are employed for scintillation imaging. Potential radionuclide impurities in Tl-201 include Pb-203, Tl-200, and Tl-202. At the time of calibration, Tl-201 should contain less than 0.25% Pb-203 (279 KeV), 0.3% Tl-200 (368 KeV), and no more than 1% Tl-202 (439 KeV). The level of these radionuclidic contaminants is critical, since downscatter from the higher-energy photons can seriously degrade image quality.

The critical organ, the kidneys, receives approximately 2.4 rads from 2.0 mCi.

Method

Resting Study. Scintillation images are taken beginning 10 minutes after radiopharmaceutical administration. Scintillation images should be taken in anterior, 45° left anterior oblique (LAO), and left lateral (or 70° LAO) projections (Fig. 15–4).

Exercise Stress Study. A catheter line is

Table 15–4.   Interpretation of myocardial perfusion imaging studies.

Results of Exercise Image	Results of Rest Image	Clinical Interpretation
Normal	Normal	No clinically significant coronary artery disease
Abnormal	Normal	Stress-induced myocardial ischemia
Abnormal	Abnormal	Myocardial infarction
Additional abnormal area(s)	Abnormal	Myocardial infarction with areas of stress-induced myocardial ischemia

A.   Tl-203 (p, 3n) Pb-201

B. $Pb\text{-}201 \xrightarrow[T\frac{1}{2} = 9.4 \text{ hr}]{EC} Tl\text{-}201$

Fig. 15–3.   (A) Production of Pb-201 and (B) its decay to Tl-201.

placed into a peripheral vein, the patient is stressed to the desired level (using treadmill or ergometer), and the Tl-201 thallous chloride is administered. To ensure adequate distribution of the radiopharmaceutical the patient continues exercising for at least 30 seconds after administration of Tl-201 thallous chloride. Imaging is started within 3 to 10 minutes and finished by 30 minutes (Fig. 15–5). Delayed images (at rest) are also obtained approximately one hour after completion of stress imaging.

Special Considerations/Patient Preparation

The apex of the heart usually concentrates much less Tl-201 than other parts of the myocardium and may appear as an area of faint uptake. Absence of Tl-201 activity in the aortic outflow region of the LAO view is entirely normal, and the atria are rarely visualized. Physiologic motion artifacts can be controlled, to an extent, by using gated imaging techniques. Also, computer-assisted circumferential profile analysis of Tl-201 images can be helpful in providing standardized, quantitative evaluation of myocardial perfusion. Submaximal exercise substantially diminishes the sensitivity of the Tl-201 stress test.

In order to reduce the uptake of Tl-201 by the viscera, patients should be NPO.

While it is known that potassium transport is affected by alterations in blood glucose, insulin, and pH (as in diabetes mellitus), no data is currently available to substantiate any effect of these conditions on Tl-201 distribution.

Interventional Agents

Dipyridamole, a potent coronary arteriolar vasodilator, can be used during Tl-201 thallous chloride myocardial scintigraphy to increase normal coronary blood flow in order to detect areas of myocardium affected by stenosed vessels (which do not respond to dipyridamole). Dipyridamole/Tl-201 thallous chloride scintigraphy has been primarily employed in patients unable to exercise to their ischemic threshold as a substitute for the standard exercise treadmill study. Typically, the technique is to infuse the supine patient with dipyridamole intravenously over several minutes

Table 15–5.   Nuclear properties of Tl-201.

	Decay Mode	Physical Half-life	Principal Photons	
			Energy	Yield
Tl-201	EC	73.1 hr	68–80 KeV (Hg x rays)	95%
			135 KeV	2.7%
			167 KeV	10.0%

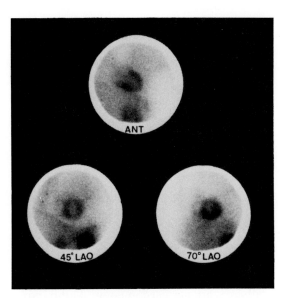

Fig. 15–4. ^{201}Tl-thallous chloride study in patient with no evidence of myocardial perfusion abnormalities.

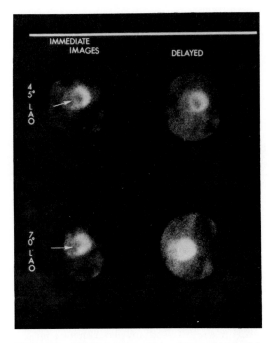

Fig. 15–5. Tl-201 images obtained immediately following exercise and images taken 1 hour later. The perfusion defect seen immediately after exercise (*arrows*) "fills" during delayed imaging and most likely represents reversible ischemia (see Table 15–4).

prior to the injection of Tl-201. Imaging, in the standard views, is immediately performed; redistribution images are obtained 3 to 4 hours later.

15.4 STUDIES OF CARDIAC FUNCTION USING BLOOD POOL RADIOPHARMACEUTICALS

Principle

The second category of heart studies, *determining cardiac function,* is performed with radiolabeled blood components or radiopharmaceuticals that remain in the blood pool. These radiolabeled substances, when imaged with sophisticated computer acquisition and image processing systems, provide diagnostic information on cardiac function. Although several radiopharmaceuticals have been used for these studies, the current agents of choice are Tc-99m–labeled autologous red blood cells and ^{99m}Tc-human serum albumin (HSA). Because of the relative convenience and reliability of Tc-99m labeling of red blood cells, ^{99m}Tc-red blood cells are usually preferred over ^{99m}Tc-human serum albumin. Some cardiac studies require only short-term retention in the blood pool (dynamic flow-type studies) and can be performed using ^{99m}Tc-sodium pertechnetate.

Indication

Measurements of cardiac function, commonly called multi-gated acquisition studies, are useful for evaluating cardiac function, including measurement of cardiac output, ejection fraction, and wall motion. This technique is also useful in the evaluation of patients with suspected cardiac disease and in following the treatment of coronary artery disease and other cardiomyopathies.

Radiopharmaceutical Data

Red blood cells may be labeled with Tc-99m either by in vitro or in vivo incubation

(A) In vivo Method	(B) In vivo/In vitro method
Step 1—Inject stannous pyrophosphate. *Step 2*—Wait approximately 20 minutes, then inject (IV) 20–25 mCi ^{99m}Tc-sodium pertechnetate.	*Step 1*—Inject (IV) stannous pyrophosphate. *Step 2*—Wait approximately 20 minutes. *Step 3*—Withdraw (via venipuncture) approximately 8 ml whole blood into a shielded syringe containing 20–25 mCi ^{99m}Tc-sodium pertechnetate.* Gently mix at room temperature for 10 minutes. *Step 4*—Reinject contents of syringe.

*Syringe may be heparinized with *very* dilute solution (10 units/ml) or contain ACD (acid-citrate-dextrose) as anticoagulant.

Fig. 15–6. Tc-99m labeling of red blood cells by the (A) in vivo method and (B) modified in vivo/in-vitro method.

of Tc-99m (as ^{99m}Tc-sodium pertechnetate) with whole blood that has been pretreated with stannous (Sn^{+2}) ions (Fig. 15–6). Stannous ion pretreatment involves the intravenous administration of stannous ions (usually in the form of stannous pyrophosphate) at a dose of 10 to 20 µg per kg body weight. Thus, stannous pyrophosphate, when labeled with Tc-99m, is the commonly employed bone and myocardial infarct imaging agent, but when injected in the nonradioactive ("cold") form, stannous pyrophosphate sensitizes RBCs for subsequent tagging with Tc-99m.

Tc-99m incubation with sensitized red blood cells can occur either by direct intravenous injection of ^{99m}Tc-sodium pertechnetate at 20 minutes following stannous pyrophosphate injection (in vivo method) or by withdrawal of a sample of stannous ion–pretreated whole blood into a shielded syringe containing ^{99m}Tc-sodium pertechnetate (in vivo/in vitro method). With either technique, usually not less than 85% of ^{99m}Tc-sodium pertechnetate labels red blood cells.

While small amounts of a dilute solution of heparin can be used as an anticoagulant

in the in vivo/in vitro method, care should be exercised to ensure that heparinized catheters are not used in either method for the administration of stannous pyrophosphate or in the in vivo method for the injection of ^{99m}Tc-sodium pertechnetate. Whenever heparinized catheters are used, inferior image quality as well as increased renal and urinary activity often results.

While it is the stannous ions that are responsible for Tc-99m labeling of RBCs, simple salts of stannous ions cannot be used because of their inherent insolubility at physiologic pH. As the chelated pyrophosphate form, however, stannous ions are sufficiently soluble yet only weakly bound to pyrophosphate. When stannous pyrophosphate is placed in contact with whole blood, stannous ions readily dissociate from pyrophosphate and complex RBCs for subsequent labeling.

The radiation dosimetry for Tc-99m–labeled red blood cells is shown in Table 15–6.

Method

Computerized data acquisition and image processing are essential components

Table 15–6. Absorbed radiation doses* (rads/20 mCi) when ^{99m}Tc-sodium pertechnetate is given 30 minutes after stannous pyrophosphate.

Bladder Wall	Stomach Wall	Ovaries	Testes	Blood	Red Marrow
0.54	1.6	0.42	0.24	1.06	0.46

*Assuming 85% Tc-99m tag to red blood cells; resting subject.

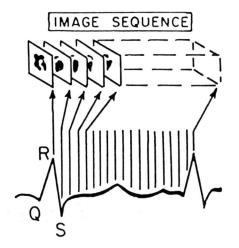

Fig. 15–7. Computer imaging sequence for EKG gated blood pool ventriculography. The sequence is normally triggered by the R wave, with the cardiac cycle divided into discrete components. Counts arriving during any division are placed in the computer matrix relevant to that division. After several hundred cardiac cycles, there is enough information on each frame to form a useful image. (From Mettler, FA, Jr., Guiberteau, MJ: Essentials of Nuclear Medicine Imaging. New York, Grune and Stratton, 1983.)

for nuclear studies of cardiac function (Fig. 15–7).

Special Considerations/Patient Preparation

Patients should be NPO in order to avoid any altered blood flow to the nearby liver.

REFERENCES

1. Berne, RM, Levy, MN: Cardiovascular Physiology. St. Louis, C.V. Mosby Co., 1977.
2. Bonte, FJ, Parkey, RW: A new method for myocardial infarct imaging. J Nucl Med 15:479–485, 1974.
3. Callahan, RJ, Froelich, JW, McKusick, KA, et al.: A modified method for the in-vivo labeling of red blood cells with Tc-99m: concise communication. J Nucl Med 23:315–318, 1982.
4. Chervu, LR: Radiopharmaceuticals in cardiovascular nuclear medicine. Semin Nucl Med 9:241–256, 1979.
5. Dewanjee, MK: Cardiac and vascular imaging with labeled platelets and leukocytes. Semin Nucl Med 14(3):154–187, July 1984.
6. Hegge, FN, Hamilton, GW, Larson, SM, et al.: Cardiac chamber imaging: a comparison of red blood cells labeled with ^{99m}Tc in vitro and in vivo. J Nucl Med 19:129–134, 1978.
7. Kirchner, PT (ed.): Nuclear Medicine Review Syllabus. New York, Society of Nuclear Medicine, 1980, pp. 103–158.
8. Pierson, RN, Jr, Friedman, MI, Tansey, WA, et al.: Cardiovascular nuclear medicine: an overview. Semin Nucl Med 9:224–240, 1979.
9. Porter, WC, Dees, SM, Frietas, JE, et al.: Acid-citrate-dextrose compared with heparin in the preparation of in vivo/in vitro technetium-99m red blood cells. J Nucl Med, 24:383–387, 1983.
10. Smith, TD, Richard P: A simple kit for the preparation of ^{99m}Tc-labeled red blood cells. J Nucl Med 17:126–132, 1976.
11. Stokely, EM, Parkey, RW, Bonte, FR, et al.: Gated blood imaging following Tc-99, stannous pyrophosphate imaging. J Nucl Med 120:433–434, 1976.
12. Strauss, HW, Pitt, B: Thallium-201 as a myocardial imaging agent. Semin Nucl Med 7:49–58, 1977.

Radiopharmaceuticals for Pulmonary Imaging

16.1 PULMONARY IMAGING

Although pulmonary arterial blood supply can be accurately imaged by arteriography, this is an invasive procedure that is relatively expensive, requires experienced personnel, and cannot be conveniently performed in an emergency. Nuclear medicine studies of lung, on the other hand, are very sensitive indicators of pulmonary function and can be conveniently performed with relatively little risk. For these reasons, nuclear medicine procedures are often first-line studies in the investigation of pulmonary disease.

Nuclear medicine studies of lung can be divided into two categories—studies of *regional pulmonary perfusion* with radiolabeled particles, and studies of *lung ventilation function* using either radioactive gases or radioaerosols.

16.2 REGIONAL PULMONARY PERFUSION IMAGING

Principle

When radiolabeled particles larger than red blood cells are administered intravenously, they become trapped within the capillary beds of the lung. Provided these radiolabeled particles are mixed homogeneously in blood in the right side of the heart and are almost entirely extracted in lung during first passage, their appearance in the lung will provide images of regional pulmonary perfusion. Areas not perfused will appear as "cold" areas (Fig. 16–1).

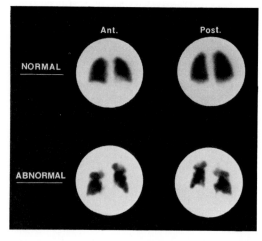

Fig. 16–1. Normal perfusion lung study vs abnormal perfusion study. Both studies were performed with ^{99m}Tc-macroaggregated albumin (MAA); (note the nonperfused "cold" areas, which are devoid of radioactivity in the abnormal perfusion study).

Indications

The primary indication for pulmonary perfusion imaging is to screen for pulmonary emboli (changes in pulmonary perfusion, however, are not limited to pulmonary emboli and can result from other types of lung diseases, such as emphysema, bronchitis, and asthma).

Radiopharmaceutical Data

Several radiopharmaceuticals have been employed for pulmonary perfusion imaging, including radiolabeled iron hydroxide particles and macroaggregates of human serum albumin labeled with either I-131 or Tc-99m. Presently, ^{99m}Tc-macroaggregated albumin (MAA) and ^{99m}Tc-labeled human albumin microspheres (HAM) are the agents of choice for pulmonary perfusion imaging.

Both ^{99m}Tc-MAA and ^{99m}Tc-HAM are prepared from human serum albumin that has been heat-denatured in either an acidified water bath (MAA) or oil (HAM). Differences between ^{99m}Tc-MAA and ^{99m}Tc-HAM particles relate to:

1. *Shape and particle size*—HAM particles are spherical and slightly more uniform in size than the irregularly shaped MAA particles.
2. *Residence time in lung*—HAM particles have slightly longer lung T½ than MAA particles (4 to 5 hr vs 2 to 3 hr).
3. *Lung clearance mechanisms*—MAA particles are cleared from lung by breakdown into smaller particles that pass through the lung and are subsequently phagocytized by cells of the RE system. Spherical HAM particles are removed from the lung after being enzymatically solubilized.

Both HAM and MAA preparations are commercially available as lyophilized kits and utilize Sn^{+2} ions for Tc-99m reduction and radiolabeling. A primary difference exists between the methods of on-site preparation of these two agents: upon the addition of ^{99m}Tc-sodium pertechnetate, HAM kits must be placed into an ultrasound water bath usually for not less than 5 minutes. This step assists the coating of HAM particles by Pluronic F-68, a detergent, which acts as a surface active agent to stabilize particle size and prevent the formation of undesirably large HAM particles. MAA kits do not require this sonification step during on-site radiolabeling and preparation. The biological properties of MAA and HAM are compared in Table 16–1.

Several factors, including the size and number of injected particles, have been shown to affect image quality and patient safety.

For example, the injection of particles much larger than the diameters of the precapillary arterioles (Table 16–2) yield no greater diagnostic information and may prove harmful because the particles will occlude pulmonary blood flow at a much higher vascular level. On the other hand, particles much smaller than the terminal capillary units ($\cong 8$ to 9μ) will pass through the lungs and subsequently be removed by the cells of the reticuloendothelial system. To optimize image quality and prevent any likelihood of altered hemodynamics from the injection of particles larger than required, USP XXI specifies that not less than 90% of MAA or HAM particles have a diameter between 10 and 90μ and none of the particles have a diameter greater than 150μ.

The number of MAA or HAM particles injected is also important. The injection of too few ^{99m}Tc-MAA or -HAM particles, for example, can result in apparent perfusion defects in normal patients, because the random distribution of a small number of particles produces an uneven appearance of the radiopharmaceutical in the lung. This is particularly true today because of the improved resolution of newer scintillation cameras. For this reason, it is suggested that adult patients receive no less than

Table 16–1.   Comparison of biologic ^{99m}Tc-human albumin microspheres (HAM) and ^{99m}Tc-macroaggregated albumin (MAA).

	^{99m}Tc MAA	^{99m}Tc HAM
Particle size range (microns)	10–50	10–35
Biologic T½ (lungs)	2–3 hr	4–5 hr
Lung clearance mechanism	Fragmentation	Enzymatic dissolution
Range of number of particles per vial in commercially available products	1.0–8.0×10^6	$\cong 1 \times 10^6$

Table 16–2. The pulmonary vasculature.

Vessel	Number in Adult Lung	Approximate Diameter (Microns)
Distribution artery connectors	0.25×10^6	135
Distribution arteries	4×10^6	60–100
Precapillary arterioles	300×10^6	30
Terminal capillary units	280×10^9	8

60,000–100,000 HAM or MAA particles. Although the use of much larger numbers of particles ($>10^6$) has been shown to produce no appreciable changes in pulmonary hemodynamics, it is advisable that patient doses contain not more than 2×10^6 particles, since any larger number would unnecessarily occlude pulmonary capillaries (Table 16–2). Ideally, an adult dose should contain 100,000–500,000 particles.

Dosages for pediatric patients, on the other hand, should contain significantly fewer particles since lung capillary beds are not fully developed for some time after birth. If 500,000 particles are considered safe for adults, it has been estimated that newborns should receive no more than 50,000 particles, and one-year-olds, less than 165,000 particles.

Although antigenic reactions have been reported in patients receiving these radiopharmaceuticals, the overall incidence is very low.

Methods

The usual adult dose of either ^{99m}Tc-MAA or ^{99m}Tc-HAM is 3 to 5 mCi. During injection, patients should be supine since gravitational effects on blood flow in patients injected either standing or sitting can cause an uneven distribution of particles, with a greater part of the radiopharmaceutical dose appearing at the base of the lungs. Since localization of these particles in lung is rapid, scintillation images may be obtained immediately after injection. Usually a minimum of six lung views—anterior, posterior, right and left lateral, and right and left posterior obliques—are obtained.

Special Considerations/Patient Preparation

No patient preparation is required.

During injection of either ^{99m}Tc-MAA or -HAM, syringes that have contained blood for more than a few seconds should be discarded, since blood clots formed containing the radiopharmaceutical would appear as "hot" spots during lung imaging.

Special consideration should also be given to the number of particles administered (particularly in newborns and children) and to the patient's position during injection. These factors have been previously discussed.

The primary contraindication to pulmonary perfusion imaging is severe pulmonary hypertension. Care should also be exercised in the use of these radiopharmaceuticals in patients suspected of right-to-left cardiac shunts.

16.3 PULMONARY VENTILATION IMAGING

Principle

While pulmonary perfusion imaging is a very sensitive indicator of abnormalities in lung blood supply, it frequently lacks the specificity necessary to distinguish pulmonary emboli from other types of lung disease (such as asthma and obstructive lung diseases) that also produce perfusion defects. Greater diagnostic specificity usually results when studies of lung ventila-

Table 16–3. Match/mismatch of perfusion and ventilation imaging for the differentiation of pulmonary emboli from obstructive-type lung diseases.

	Perfusion Study	Ventilation Study*
Pulmonary emboli	Abnormal	Normal
Chronic-type obstructive lung diseases (emphysema, asthma, etc.)	Abnormal	Abnormal

*During ventilation imaging, areas of lung affected by *pulmonary emboli* usually have normal ventilation patterns. Ventilation imaging in patients with *chronic-type obstructive lung disease* shows affected areas as very slow to fill during the radioactive gas single breath-hold phase. These areas eventually fill in during equilibrium. Later, during the radiogas washout phase, these same areas demonstrate gas trapping in the affected region.

tion are performed in conjunction with abnormal perfusion imaging (Table 16–3).

Indications

Pulmonary ventilation imaging is indicated in the assessment of possible pulmonary emboli and regional pulmonary function.

Radiopharmaceutical Data

Presently, the radioactive gases, Xe-127 and Xe-133, are the agents most commonly employed for ventilation imaging. Kr-81m, a generator-produced radionuclide, is also useful for ventilation imaging. A comparison of the relative properties of these radiopharmaceuticals is shown in Table 16–4.

In the majority of clinical situations it is preferable to perform ventilation imaging following abnormal 99mTc-MAA/HAM perfusion studies. With Xe-133, however, this is not always possible, since the scatter to lower energies of Tc-99m photons from the previously administered radiopharmaceutical have very nearly the same energy as the principal photons of Xe-133. Therefore they cannot be readily distinguished from Xe-133 (Fig. 16–2). For this reason, Xe-133 ventilation imaging is often performed either immediately before the 99mTc-MAA/HAM perfusion study or on the following day. The higher energy principal photons of Xe-127, however, permit ventilation imaging to be performed immediately following Tc-99m perfusion imaging without image degradation. Also, since the perfusion study is performed first, the follow-up Xe-127 ventilation study can be performed with the patient in a position that allows optimal visualization of the previously noted perfusion defect.

Since xenon is physiologically inert, the relatively long physical half-lives of Xe-133 (5.27 days) and Xe-127 (36.4 days) do not contribute significantly to patient radiation exposure. In fact, largely because of its electron capture decay mode, Xe-127 provides a substantially lower patient radiation dose than does Xe-133 (which decays by β$^-$ emission). Like Xe-127, Kr-81m also has higher principal photon energies, which enables ventilation imaging to be

Table 16–4. Physical properties of radiopharmaceuticals used in lung ventilation imaging.

Radionuclide	Decay Mode	Physical T½	Principal Photons	
			Energy (KeV)	Abundance (%)
Xe-133	β$^-$	5.3 days	81	35
Xe-127	EC	36.4 days	172	68
			203	25
Kr-81m*	EC	13 sec	190	65

*[Rb-81 → Kr-81m]
T½ = 4.7 hr

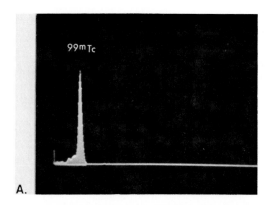

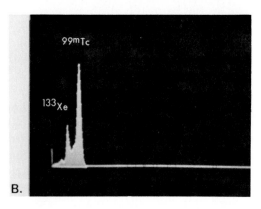

Fig. 16–2. (A) Pulse-height spectra of Tc-99m and (B) of both Tc-99m *and* Xe-133. Note that the principal photopeak of Xe-133 lies in the Compton scatter region of Tc-99m. This can make it difficult to separate the photopeaks of these two radionuclides in clinical studies when Tc-99m is used first. Although equal activities were used to prepare these pulse-height spectra, the lower Xe-133 peak reflects its lower photon abundance.

performed immediately after Tc-99m perfusion imaging. Kr-81m also decays by electron capture and provides relatively minimal radiation exposure to the patient.

Method

Ventilation studies with radioactive xenon are usually performed with the assistance of a shielded, closed spirometer system. The radioactive gas is administered by inhalation, with the xenon ventilation study divided into three phases (1) *initial single breath-hold* (or "wash-in"), (2) *radiogas equilibrium*, and (3) *radiogas wash-*

out. The study commences with the bolus administration of xenon into the lungs; usually, 15 to 20 mCi of Xe-133 or 5 to 10 mCi of Xe-127 is employed (Fig.16–3). With the bolus administration technique, the patient holds his or her breath as long as comfortably possible while the image (i.e., the "single breath-hold image") is obtained. Following this initial image, successive images are also obtained (usually over 30-second intervals) for approximately 3 to 5 minutes as the radiogas concentration in the lungs and the breathing apparatus approaches equilibrium. Later, images of radiogas washout from lungs are also obtained as the patient breathes room air. Images obtained during radiogas washout from lung are very sensitive indicators of lung trapping abnormalities such as occur in chronic-type lung diseases (Fig. 16–4). During radiogas washout, the expired xenon must be either vented from the room in accordance with NRC (or state regulatory agency) regulations or trapped in a shielded gas trapping device.

Kr-81m, a generator-produced radionuclide, is administered directly from a ^{81}Rb-^{81m}Kr generator. Unlike with the radioxenons, however, the ultrashort physical half-life of Kr-81m prevents radiogas equilibrium and washout imaging during ventilation. For this reason, images of Kr-81m distribution reflect regional ventilation. A major disadvantage to Kr-81m is that its parent, Rb-81, has a 4.7-hour physical half-life, which limits generator usefulness to one day only and necessitates relatively expensive air freight deliveries. The 13-second physical half-life of Kr-81m is advantageous for disposal, however, since expired Kr-81m can be exhausted directly into the room without the need for a trapping device.

16.4   XENON-IN-SALINE— PERFUSION/VENTILATION IMAGING

Although xenon is only slightly soluble in water, it is sufficiently soluble to allow

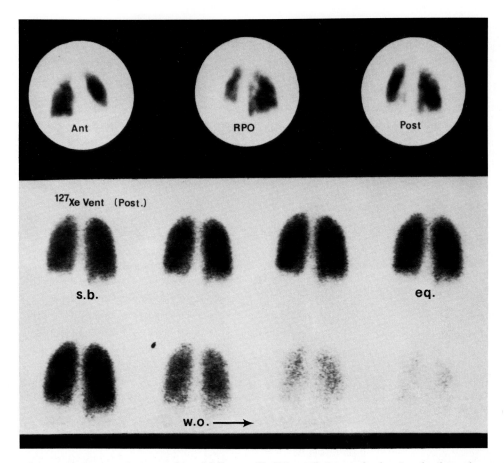

Fig. 16–3. ^{99m}Tc-MAA perfusion study and follow-up Xe-127 ventilation study showing the three phases of ventilation imaging: initial single breath image (s.b.), radiogas equilibrium (eq.), and radiogas washout (w.o.). Diagnosis is most likely pulmonary emboli, since the perfusion study shows multiple abnormalities that do not appear during radiogas ventilation. See Table 16–3.

the preparation of xenon-saline solutions, which can be administered intravenously. Approximately 95% of the injected xenon in saline is cleared from blood into the lungs during the first pass. For this reason an immediate scintillation image of the xenon-133 distribution in lung depicts pulmonary blood flow, while later sequential images demonstrate radiogas clearance from the lungs. There are some disadvantages to this technique. First, the poor solubility of xenon makes handling and injection of this agent difficult. Second, because of the rapid clearance of the radiopharmaceutical from blood only one view of perfusion can be obtained. Third, since in the U.S. there are at present no

commercial suppliers of xenon-saline solutions, this agent must be prepared in-house from xenon gas and saline.

16.5 RADIOLABELED AEROSOLS

Recently there has been renewed interest in the use of radioaerosols as an alternative to radiogas ventilation imaging. These agents are prepared by placing either ^{99m}Tc-DTPA, ^{99m}Tc-sulfur colloid, or other commonly available radiopharmaceuticals into commercially available nebulizers. When the radioaerosol technique was first introduced during the mid-1960s, problems with control and uniformity of particle size resulted in the formation of

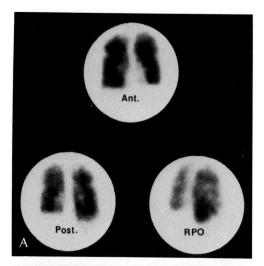

Fig. 16–4. (A) Lung perfusion study demonstrating multiple perfusion abnormalities and (B) ^{127}Xe ventilation study showing corresponding gas trapping in the involved areas *(arrows)*. This patient was diagnosed as having chronic-type lung disease with only a low probability of pulmonary emboli.

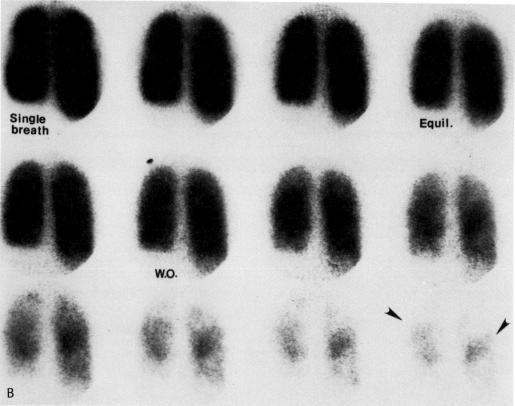

large particles that deposited in central airways, producing "hot" spots that appeared during imaging. Today, with advances in aerosol technology, this problem is essentially nonexistent.

To perform a radioaerosol lung study, the patient breathes directly from a nebulizer that contains 30 to 45 mCi of the Tc-99m radiopharmaceutical. Usually less than 2% of the radioactivity is deposited in lungs as the patient breathes the radioaerosol for 3 to 5 minutes. The patient is immediately imaged at the end of this period and, since most radiopharmaceuticals have a biological half-life in the lungs of approximately 1.0 hour, multiple views can be obtained.

Clinically, the value of radiolabeled aerosols in the diagnosis of lung airway disease is well established, although the use of Tc-99m as a radiolabel for *both* the perfusion and radioaerosol agents makes it difficult to perform perfusion/aerosol imaging on the same day.

REFERENCES

1. Alderson, PO, Riyannavech, N, Secker-Walker, RH, et al.: The role of Xe-133 ventilation studies in the scintigraphic detection of pulmonary embolism. Radiology 120:633–640, 1976.
2. Alpert, NM, McKusick, KA, Correia, JA, et al.: Initial assessment of a simple functional image of ventilation. J Nucl Med 17:83–92, 1976.
3. Atkins, HL, Susskind, H, Klopper, JF, et al.: A clinical comparison of Xe-127 and Xe-133 for ventilation studies . J Nucl Med 18:653–659, 1977.
4. Carey, JE, Purdy, JM, Moses, DC: Localization of Xe-133 in liver during ventilation studies. J Nucl Med 15:1179–1181, 1974.
5. Chilton, HM, Cooper, JF, Friedman, BI: [127]Xe ventilation imaging immediately following ^{99m}Tc perfusion studies. Clin Nucl Med 2:152–154, 1977.
6. Goris, ML, Daspit, SG, Walter, JP, et al.: Applications of ventilation lung imaging with [81m]Krypton. Radiology 122:399–403, 1977.
7. Harding, LK, Horsfield, K, Singhal, SS: Proportion of lung vessels blocked by albumin microspheres. J Nucl Med 14:579–581, 1973.
8. Heck, LL, Duley, JW: Statistical considerations in lung imaging with Tc-99m albumin particles. Radiology 113:657–679, 1974.
9. Levine, G, Malhi, B: Theoretical considerations in the preparation of Tc-99m MAA for pulmonary perfusion studies. J Nucl Med Tech 9:37–39, 1981.
10. Levine, G: A model for administering the desired number of particles for pulmonary perfusion studies. J Nucl Med Tech 8:33–36, 1980.
11. McNeil, BJ: A diagnostic strategy using ventilation-perfusion studies in patients suspect for pulmonary embolism. J Nucl Med 17:613–616, 1976.
12. Susskind, H, Atkins, HL, Goldman, AG, et al.: Sensitivity of Kr-81m and Xe-127 in evaluating nonembolic pulmonary disease. J Nucl Med 22:781–786, 1981.
13. Taplin, GV, Poe, ND, Dore, EK, et al.: Radioaerosol inhalation scanning. *In* Pulmonary Investigation and Radionuclides. Edited by AJ Gilson, W Smoak. Springfield, Charles C Thomas, 1970, p. 296.

CHAPTER 17

Therapeutic Applications of Radiopharmaceuticals

Radiopharmaceuticals used for therapy (Table 17–1) are designed to deliver relatively high doses of radiation to selected target tissues while producing acceptable levels of damage to nearby organs or tissues. For therapeutic agents, beta emission is preferable since the radiation dose is largely confined to target tissues and will not pose any significant external radiation hazard to nursing staff or family members. In some cases, however, radiopharmaceuticals with both beta and gamma emissions may be desirable since gamma emissions may be used for imaging in order to determine whether desired localization of the therapeutic agent has been achieved.

The radiation dose should be delivered quickly, with most of the radiopharmaceutical localizing in target tissues soon after administration. Occasionally, where target uptake may be slowed or prohibited by standard administration techniques (i.e., IV, PO), it may be desirable to place the radiopharmaceutical directly into the target tissue (e.g., via intracavitary instillation).

17.1 TREATMENT OF THYROID DISEASE WITH ¹³¹I-SODIUM IODIDE

¹³¹I-sodium iodide provides a convenient and effective method for the treatment of hyperthyroidism and some forms of thyroid cancer. Following oral administration,

I-131 is rapidly absorbed, removed from blood, and concentrated in the thyroid follicles. About 95% of the radiation dose from I-131 is delivered to the follicular epithelium by locally absorbed beta emissions that have a maximum range in tissue of approximately 2 mm. This selective irradiation of thyroid cells causes cessation of cell division, eventual cell death, and loss of thyroid hormone production. Depending upon the amount of I-131 administered, the extent of loss of thyroid function (i.e., therapy) can be controlled and a desired response obtained.

17.2 I-131 TREATMENT OF HYPERTHYROIDISM (GRAVES' DISEASE)

Prior to the treatment with I-131 of a thyrotoxic patient, the following questions must be answered:

1. What is the mass of the thyroid gland?
2. What radiation dose is necessary for the desired treatment response?
3. What is the effective half-life of I-131 in the thyroid gland?

Estimation of thyroid mass is critical, since the amount of I-131 that must be administered relates to the amount of tissue to be treated. Various techniques to measure gland size have been proposed, though most experienced clinicians still rely on physical examination.

Table 17–1.   Therapeutic radiopharmaceuticals and their indications.

Therapeutic Application	Radiopharmaceutical	Decay Mode	Administration Route
Thyroid cancer, metastatic thyroid cancer, and hyperthyroidism	^{131}I-sodium iodide	β^-,γ	PO
Polycythemia vera	^{32}P-sodium phosphate	β^-	IV
Malignant effusion	^{32}P-chromic phosphate	β^-	Intracavitary instillation

Decisions regarding the amount of radiation dose to be delivered focus on the extent of thyroid treatment desired. While there are some variations in treatment strategies, the formula of Silver (below) is one method used to determine the I-131 activity necessary to control thyrotoxicosis.

A_0 = Activity of I-131 administered (mCi)

$$A_0 = \frac{\text{Desired radiation dose (rads)} \times \text{Thyroid weight (grams)}}{\% \ 24 \text{ hour uptake}^* \times 900}$$

Generally, in the treatment of hyperthyroidism, administered I-131 activities must be sufficient to provide thyroid doses around 16,000 rads (± 2000).

While the effective half-life of radioiodine in hyperthyroidism can vary significantly, published data suggest mean values of 5.2 to 5.9 days, with individual values of 2 to 8 days. Silver's formula assumes a 6-day effective half-life.

17.3 I-131 TREATMENT OF THYROID CARCINOMA

Patients with high-risk papillary carcinoma and follicular carcinoma are primary candidates for I-131 therapy. For ablation of thyroid tissues, up to 200 mCi of I-131 may be necessary to deliver the necessary 50,000–60,000 rads. Metastatic lesions may be identified by whole body imaging with small (2 mCi) activities of I-131 (Fig. 17–1). These lesions are also treated with I-131 during the course of thyroid treatment.

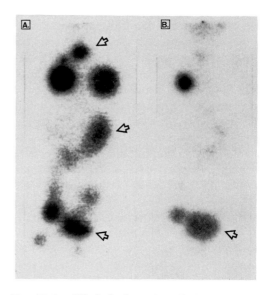

Fig. 17–1.   Whole body metastatic surveys performed with 2.0 mCi ^{131}I-sodium iodide. Image A was performed prior to I-131 oral therapy. *Arrows* indicate areas of normal I-131 excretion and distribution (thyroid, stomach, and bladder). Other areas of I-131 uptake occur in metastatic lesions involving chest nodes, lung, and bone. The patient was treated with 200 mCi of I-131, and a whole body survey was performed several months later. This study (Image B) showed a marked difference in radiopharmaceutical distribution. Specifically, abnormal uptake occurred only in the lung lesion.

Because large amounts of I-131 are used in the treatment of thyroid cancer, other body tissues receive sizeable radiation doses. For example, a 100-mCi dose of ^{131}I-sodium iodide delivers 38 rads to the red marrow. Ultimately, in patients receiving large amounts of I-131, bone marrow function may be depressed, a factor that limits their treatment with I-131. During therapy, complete blood counts should be obtained routinely.

*% uptake is expressed as whole number (i.e., 45% = 45).

17.4 PROTOCOL FOR I-131 THERAPY

Patients receiving less than 30 mCi of I-131 are not required to be hospitalized, while patients receiving more than 30 mCi must be hospitalized for radiation safety precautions until their body burden is less than this amount. During hospitalization, patients should be kept in private rooms and allowed only minimal visitation. Toilets should be flushed twice after use, and any excreta not disposed of by sanitary sewer system should be carefully contained for proper disposal by members of the institution's health protection group. Patients being discharged are instructed to be meticulous in their personal hygiene. Since I-131 is secreted in saliva, patients should avoid kissing anyone, especially young children, for several days afterwards.

When not contraindicated, patient pretreatment with propranolol may be useful to provide relief of symptomatic catecholamine release.

Additionally, personnel involved in dispensing or administering I-131 may be required to undergo thyroid bioassay for I-131 (see Section 19.7).

17.5 RISKS FROM THERAPEUTIC PROCEDURES

The risks of any sort of therapeutic procedure must be compared to the potential benefits for a particular patient. Therapy using high doses of ionizing radiations, just as with drugs and surgery, carries with it some risk. The possible risk from such *high* doses of radiation are generally well known and include cancer induction, organ and tissue destruction (thyroid, bone marrow, etc.), effects on the embryo/fetus, and genetic effects.

^{131}I-sodium iodide was introduced for the treatment of *hyperthyroidism* in 1942 and since about 1950 has been widely accepted as a successful means of controlling the disease. Patients treated number in the hundreds of thousands. Possible hazards involve the potential for the induction of thyroiditis and hypothyroidism.

Radiation thyroiditis is an acute condition that occurs within 2 weeks after exposure to radiation and is characterized by inflammation and eventual necrosis of some or all thyroid cells. Clinically significant radiation thyroiditis is highly unlikely at thyroid radiation doses below 20,000 rads.

Hypothyroidism occurs with Graves' disease even after surgery and has a cumulative incidence of about 20% in 10 years. Long-term incidence of hypothyroidism after I-131 therapy seems to depend upon the amount of radioactivity administered, with the cumulative incidence over 10 years varying between 30 and 70%.

Since iodine crosses the placenta, treatment with I-131 of thyrotoxicosis in pregnant patients beyond 10 weeks gestation has resulted in *hypothyroid children*. For this reason, I-131 therapy should not be used during pregnancy. Use of pregnancy tests is highly recommended in potentially pregnant patients who are to receive therapeutic levels of I-131.

Treatment of hyperthyroid patients with 10 mCi of I-131 provides a radiation dose to ovaries or testes of less than 3 rads. Since this activity is within the range given by many common diagnostic roentgenologic procedures, it seems as unreasonable to withhold I-131 treatment from young men and nonpregnant young women on grounds of *genetic hazard* alone as it would be to withhold diagnostic x-rays.

In view of the very large number of patients treated with I-131, the reported numbers of *thyroid cancers* certainly does not indicate an incidence in excess of chance expectations, even allowing for a long latent period (Chapter 6).

Induction of *leukemia* was considered to be a possible side effect of I-131 treatment for hyperthyroidism because of sporadic reports in the 1950s of leukemia in patients following radioiodine therapy. In 1968, the results of a cooperative study involving 18,400 patients with thyrotoxicosis treated with I-131 as compared to 10,700 treated with surgery was reported. When the incidence of leukemia in radioiodine-treated patients was compared to the incidence in surgically treated patients, no difference was demonstrated, although the incidence of leukemia in *both* groups was greater than in the population at large.

17.6 THERAPEUTIC APPLICATIONS WITH P-32 RADIOPHARMACEUTICALS

P-32 is a pure beta-emitting radionuclide (β^- energy of 1.71 MeV max.) with a 14.3-day physical half-life. P-32 can be used as the soluble sodium phosphate for the treatment of several hematologic disorders (primarily polycythemia vera) or as colloidal P-32 chromic phosphate for the treatment of malignant effusions.

17.7 TREATMENT OF POLYCYTHEMIA VERA WITH P-32 SODIUM PHOSPHATE

P-32 sodium phosphate is a *clear, colorless solution* that, upon intravenous administration, concentrates in blood cell precursors of the bone marrow at sites where there is rapid proliferation of cells. The local β^- radiation of P-32 destroys cell production capacities. A dose of 4 mCi of P-32 delivers about 100 rads to bone marrow, liver, and spleen; the remainder of the body receives about 10 rads.

It has been known since 1945 that acute leukemia occurs in polycythemia vera patients treated with P-32. Acute leukemia, however, also occurs in patients with polycythemia vera treated without radiation, using only drugs or phlebotomy. It is uncertain whether the observed incidence of leukemia following P-32 therapy is the result of therapy or of other factors. It is possible that P-32 therapy, by prolonging life, permits the natural evolution of polycythemia vera into acute leukemia, or that the possible carcinogenic action of P-32 results from irradiation of a susceptible population.

17.8 TREATMENT OF MALIGNANT EFFUSION WITH P-32 CHROMIC PHOSPHATE

P-32 chromic phosphate is a *bluish green colloidal* suspension that is instilled directly into the body cavity containing the malignant effusion. *It is never given intravenously.* After cavity instillation, the β^- radiation dose is delivered to the surface of the cavity, onto which the radioactive colloid adheres. To ensure that no loculation of the P-32 chromic phosphate occurs, ^{99m}Tc-sulfur colloid may be instilled just prior to the P-32 chromic phosphate, and scintillation images may be obtained of its distribution in the body cavity. Usually between 3 and 6 mCi of ^{32}P-chromic phosphate is administered.

REFERENCES

1. Beierwaltes, WH: The treatment of hyperthyroidism with iodine-131. Semin Nucl Med 8:95–103, 1978.
2. Beierwaltes, WH: The treatment of thyroid carcinoma with radioactive iodine. Semin Nucl Med 8:79–94, 1978.
3. Berek, PD, Goldberg, JD, Silverstein, MN, et al.: Increased incidence of acute leukemia in polycythemia vera associated with chlorambucil therapy. New Engl J Med 304:441–447, 1981.
4. Maxon, HR, Thomas, SR, Saenger, EL, et al.: Ionizing irradiation and the induction of clinically significant disease in the human thyroid gland. Am J Med 63:967–978, 1977.
5. NCRP Report No. 70. Nuclear Medicine—Factors influencing the choice and use of radionuclides in diagnosis and therapy. National Council on Radiation Protection and Measurements, Bethesda, Maryland, 1982.
6. Saenger, EL, Kereiakes, JG, Sodd, VJ, et al.: Radiotherapeutic agents: Properties, dosimetry and radiobiologic considerations. Semin Nucl Med 9:72–84, 1979.
7. NCRP Report No. 80. Induction of thyroid cancer by ionizing radiation. Bethesda, MD, National Council on Radiation Protection and Measurements, 1985.

Regulations Affecting Radiopharmaceuticals

The manufacture, distribution, possession, and use of radiopharmaceuticals are controlled by a number of federal, state, and local agencies, whose authority occasionally overlaps. This chapter provides an overview of these agencies and their primary jurisdiction and regulatory activities, along with a discussion of specific regulations that must be met in order to safely use radiopharmaceuticals.

18.1 NUCLEAR REGULATORY COMMISSION (NRC)

The NRC is the primary federal agency empowered to regulate radioactive materials. The NRC was created by the Energy Reorganization Act of 1974. This act abolished the original federal regulatory agency, the Atomic Energy Commission (AEC), and transferred to the NRC all licensing and regulatory functions originally assigned to the AEC by the Atomic Energy Act of 1954 (as amended). Specifically, the authority of the NRC is limited to regulating the possession, use, and disposal of the following types of radioactive materials:

1. Reactor by-product materials (materials produced by a nuclear reactor)
2. Special nuclear materials (U-233 or plutonium or uranium enriched with U-233 or U-235)
3. Source materials (uranium or thorium in any form).

The Atomic Energy Act of 1954, as amended, provided that individual states, by agreement with the AEC, could accept

Table 18–1. Agreement states (those that have accepted responsibility to regulate radioactive materials) and states regulated by NRC.

AGREEMENT STATES (27)	NRC (23)*
Alabama	Alaska
Arizona	Connecticut
Arkansas	Delaware
California	Hawaii
Colorado	Illinois
Florida	Indiana
Georgia	Iowa
Idaho	Maine
Kansas	Massachusetts
Kentucky	Michigan
Louisiana	Minnesota
Maryland	Missouri
Mississippi	Montana
Nebraska	New Jersey
Nevada	Ohio
New Hampshire	Oklahoma
New Mexico	Pennsylvania
New York	South Dakota
North Carolina	Vermont
North Dakota	Virginia
Oregon	West Virginia
Rhode Island	Wisconsin
South Carolina	Wyoming
Tennessee	
Texas	
Utah	
Washington	

*NRC authority also extends to several U.S. Territories and the District of Columbia.

responsibility to regulate radioactive materials as long as the state regulations were compatible with those regulations of the AEC (now NRC). Under this agreement with NRC these states (called *Agreement States*) usually are responsible for regulating the possession, use, and disposal of all radioactive materials, including naturally occurring *and* accelerator-produced radioactive materials. States subject to NRC ju-

150

risdiction usually have state-level agencies to control accelerator-produced radioactive materials. A list of agreement states and those regulated by NRC is shown in Table 18–1.

18.2 AUTHORIZATION AND LICENSURE

NRC authorization to use reactor by-product materials (or Agreement States' authorization to use by-product materials and accelerator-produced radionuclides) is generally governed by specific types of licenses. These licenses (Table 18–2) may be granted to either institutions or physicians and pharmacists, who document the required experience and training in the safe handling and use of radioactive materials. NRC has published criteria for adequate training and experience for persons seeking to possess and use radionuclides. A description of information to be included in a license application for radioactive materials is shown in Table 18–3.

The application process has been simplified by the NRC and now permits applicants for specific licenses of limited scope the option of requesting groups of radiopharmaceuticals for medical use. Applicants may request the use of an entire class of these materials rather than individual agents. These groups and their descriptive uses are shown in Table 18–4.

Following the granting of a radioactive materials license, it is the responsibility of the institution's Medical Isotopes Committee (along with the radiation safety officer) to ensure that the license is kept up-to-date and that the regulations are followed. At periodic intervals (usually every 2 to 5 years) licenses are inspected by either the NRC or the appropriate agency of Agreement State to ensure regulatory compliance.

18.3 REGULATIONS AFFECTING RADIATION IN WORKERS

The NRC (and most Agreement State agencies) has established regulations de-signed to ensure the protection of radiation workers. The current standard for the occupationally exposed worker is the maximum permitted dose (MPD), which gives specific upper limits of permitted occupational exposure. Adherence to these permitted dose ranges presumably carries good assurance that whatever risk there is will be very small (a so-called acceptable risk). The MPD levels are, in fact, based upon the concept of acceptable risk and are derived from a long experience of exposure of human beings to levels of ionizing radiation that have not demonstrated deleterious effects. Effects such as radiation-induced cataracts, infertility, and sterility are not induced by doses within the MPD. The possibility of cancer induction or genetic effects to individuals for doses under the MPD are thought to be negligible (Chapter 6).

The MPD limits specified by the NRC are based upon the recommendations of advisory groups, in particular the National Council on Radiation Protection (NCRP). The MPD values given by NRC (10 CFR, Part 20) are based upon the NCRP recommendation that an individual's average occupational radiation dose to the whole body or to other sensitive organs such as the bone marrow, gonads, and lens of the eye not exceed 5 rems per year. The MPD specified by the NRC is 1.25 rems/calendar quarter (1.25 rems $\times$ 4 calendar quarters = 5 rems). The quarterly limit can be exceeded (up to 3 rems/quarter), but the total accumulated dose of the individual must not exceed 5 $\times$ (N-18) rems, where N is the individual's age in years at his/her last birthday. Other less sensitive parts of the body, such as the hands, are permitted higher occupational dose limits (Table 18–5).

Maximum permissible levels for those under 18 are the same as for the general population—one tenth (1/10) of that permitted for occupational exposure. The NCRP restriction placed on the permissible radiation dose to pregnant women (dose

Table 18–2. Types of NRC material licenses for medical uses of by-product materials (human use).

LICENSE CATEGORY	GENERAL LICENSE		SPECIFIC LICENSE*		
			LIMITED SCOPE*		BROAD SCOPE
Name	In Vitro	In Vivo	Physicians (Private Practice)	Institutions	Type A
Permits use of radioactive materials for:	Laboratory testing by-product material in prepackaged form; total not to exceed 200 μCi of γ-emitting radionuclides listed below: ^{131}I or ^{125}I, ^{59}Fe, ^{75}Se, ^{14}C, ^{3}H, Mock ^{125}I	Human use for specified procedures and small possession limits of: ^{131}I-thyroid uptake (200 μCi max.) ^{51}Cr-red cell studies (200 μCi max.) ^{131}I or ^{125}I-HSA blood and plasma volumes (200 μCi max.) ^{58}Co or ^{60}Co B_{12} absorption (5 μCi max.)	Specific radiopharmaceuticals for specific procedures, not on hospital premises except through nuclear vans. No provision for training of physicians under this license	Specific radiopharmaceuticals for specific procedures, requires the formation of Radiation Safety Committee (see below). Provides for training of physicians; one license per institution	Large quantities and multiple types of byproduct materials; has Radiation Safety Committee (see below) to decide: user chemical and physical forms which can be used, activity, conditions of use; radiopharmaceuticals are not limited to specified use; training of physicians is possible.
Use permitted:	By clinical laboratories, hospitals, physicians, veterinarians	By physicians	By physicians specifically named on license	By or under supervision of named physician in hospital/medical center	By institutions with previous experience as limited scope specific license engaged in research in addition to diagnostic and therapeutic use. No individual user is named.
Approximate No. of licensees:	6800	1200	324	1758	113
Application Form:	NRC–483	NRC–482	NRC–313M	NRC–313M	NRC–313

NRC requires that the institution's Radiation Safety Committee evaluate all proposals for research, diagnosis, and therapeutic use of radionuclides and review the entire radiation safety program. At least three members are required (a user for each type of use authorized by the license, a member of the institutional nursing staff, a representative of the institutional management, and the radiation safety officer). (Note: Agreement States may require additional members of the Radiation Safety Committee.) The Committee meets at least quarterly.

*Nuclear pharmacies usually seek NRC licenses of the Specific License/Limited Scope type. The NRC has available a licensing guide specifically for nuclear pharmacies.

Table 18–3. Information required on an application for radioactive materials license.

1. Names of persons who will be authorized to use radioactive materials, including their training and experience in the safe handling of radioactive materials (Form NRC–313M or its equivalent)
2. List of groups of radioactive materials for which applicant wishes authorization (see Table 18–4)
3. List of radiation detection instruments, including survey instruments capable of detecting readings of 0.1 mrem/hr and as high as 1.0 mrem/hr
4. Method and frequency of instrument calibration
5. Description of available facilities and equipment
6. Procedures for ordering and receiving radioactive materials (includng procedures for safely opening packages containing radioactive materials)
7. Rules for the safe use, storage, and handling of radioactive materials
8. Emergency procedures
9. Area survey procedures
10. Methods of waste disposal.

Table 18–4. Group license for use of radiopharmaceuticals. Uses are grouped on the basis of user's training and experience, facilities and equipment needed, and radiation safety precautions required.

Group I	Diagnostic use of prepared radiopharmaceuticals used for measurement of uptake, dilution, and excretion studies (a prepared radiopharmaceutical is one that has been manufactured in the form to be administered to the patient and that has been labeled, packaged, and distributed in accordance with the manufacturer's radioactive materials license).
Group II	Diagnostic use of certain prepared radiopharmaceuticals for imaging and tumor localization.
Group III	Diagnostic use of radionuclide generators and kits for the preparation and use of radiopharmaceuticals.
Group IV	Therapeutic use of prepared radiopharmaceuticals that do not normally require patient hospitalization for radiation safety purposes.
Group V	Use of prepared radiopharmaceuticals for therapy requiring patient hospitalization for radiation safety purposes. Patients receiving I-131 for the treatment of thyroid carcinoma shall remain hospitalized until the residual activity is 30 mCi or less.
Group VI	The use of sealed or encased sources for therapy and bone mineral analyzers for diagnostic applications.

limit 0.5 rem during gestation) is also suggested by NRC.

Personnel Radiation Monitoring. The NRC requires the use of personnel radiation monitoring devices whenever:

1. a person enters a restricted area and is likely to receive a dose in any calendar quarter in excess of 25% of the MPD limits,
2. an individual under 18 years of age enters a restricted area and is likely to receive a dose in any calendar quarter in excess of 5% of the MPD limits, or
3. any person enters a High Radiation Area.

ALARA. The MPD limits are legal upper limits in each case. Based upon the concept that doses up to these limits carry with them an "acceptable risk" and that any reasonable effort to keep levels below these values would be beneficial, the NRC has recommended an operations philosophy that was given the acronym ALARA (which stands for "*as low as reasonably achievable*"). The ALARA concept requires

MPD limits to be considered ceilings and not the desired operating conditions. Under this approach, each exposure situation should be evaluated not in terms of how one might avoid exceeding MPD levels but in terms of how to achieve the lowest exposure commensurate with *reasonable* cost and effort.

It is also a requirement of the NRC (and

Table 18–5. Maximum permissible dose (NRC)*

Body Part	Rems/Calendar Quarter
Whole body; head and trunk; active blood-forming organs; lens of eye; or gonads	1.25
Hands and forearms; feet and ankles	18.75
Skin of whole body	7.5

*10 CFR Part 20

state regulatory agencies) that employers provide workers with access to radioactive materials licenses and regulations (which must be kept on hand by the licensee) and that employees provide, upon request, written reports of worker radiation exposure histories.

In areas where radioactive materials are handled, stored, or used, licensees must post notices and instructions to workers concerning inspections (Form NRC-3 or its equivalent) and standards for protection against radiation (see Chapter 19). Licensees are also required to post any violations found by the regulatory agency within two working days after their receipt, and these notices of violation must remain posted for a minimum of five working days or until action correcting the violation has been completed, whichever is longer (10 CFR Part 19). The licensee's response must also be posted accordingly.

18.4 FOOD AND DRUG ADMINISTRATION (FDA)

The FDA regulates the manufacturing, distribution, safety, and effectiveness of radiopharmaceuticals. This was not always the case. In 1963, the FDA exempted radiopharmaceuticals from all drug regulations as long as radiopharmaceutical manufacturers followed then-AEC regulations that covered radiation hazards of these drugs. During the 1960s, developments associated with radionuclide production technology and radiochemistry rapidly expanded the types of radiopharmaceuticals and their potential usefulness. Sensing the need to bring radiopharmaceutical regulations in line with those of traditional pharmaceuticals, the FDA removed (in 1971) many of its exemptions for radiopharmaceuticals and in 1975 terminated all exemptions. Thereafter, radiopharmaceuticals were placed under New Drug Regulations. Today, only radiopharmaceuticals that hold approved New Drug Applications (NDAs) may be distributed

commercially in the U.S., and radioactive materials with potential usefulness as radiopharmaceuticals must be investigated in accordance with FDA regulations.

Generally, the clinical investigation of a new drug is obtained in three phases:

Phase I—Pharmacology studies in a small number of persons, under carefully controlled circumstances. These studies are used to determine toxicity, metabolism, absorption, elimination, and pharmacological action (if any).

Phase II—Initial studies conducted on a limited number of patients for a specific disease or condition.

Phase III—Extensive clinical studies intended to assess the drug's safety and effectiveness and the dosage necessary in diagnosing or treating a specific disease or condition.

FDA regulations also permit the noninvestigational study of radiolabeled drugs for the evaluation of pharmacokinetic data (distribution, absorption, metabolism, and excretion only) in up to 30 patients. In this type of study the radiolabeled drug *cannot* be used for diagnostic or therapeutic purposes and the protocol must be approved by the institution's Radiopharmaceutical Drug Research Committee (RDRC). This committee is composed of persons experienced with radioactive materials and medicine as well as lay persons from the community. The composition of this committee must be approved by FDA.

In the early days of nuclear medicine, regulatory agencies exercised little control over the radiation dose to the patient. The FDA now has regulations that require calculation of patient radiation doses for investigational radiopharmaceuticals. Specifically, the regulations state that the critical organ must receive no more than 3 rems for a single dose and less than 5 rems total in a given year for limited research studies. The FDA has not issued guidelines for the practice of *clinical* nuclear medicine. The selection of appropriate activity is left to the physician, within the ALARA philosophy.

FDA and Nuclear Pharmacies. When the FDA decided in 1975 to include radiopharmaceuticals under its regulatory jurisdiction, it recognized that the unique practice of nuclear pharmacy left unsettled basic questions concerning the preparation and dispensing of these agents. Specifically, it appeared to the FDA that necessary on-site compounding of radiopharmaceuticals by combining short-lived radionuclides and reagent kits might in some situations represent drug manufacture rather than traditional pharmacy practice. In order to resolve these types of questions and better understand the nature of the practice of nuclear pharmacy, a subcommittee of the FDA's Radiopharmaceutical Advisory Committee was appointed. Its findings, which were largely supported by the FDA in its 1984 document "Nuclear Pharmacy Guidelines: Criteria for Determining When to Register as a Drug Establishment," evaluated task-analyses of nuclear pharmacies and supported the specialty practice as being within traditional state and local regulatory domain. In particular, the FDA concluded that "if the radioactive drug was prepared and dispensed under a prescription, the laws and regulations governing the practice of pharmacy and medicine at the state level should apply and the nuclear pharmacy should be considered as engaging in the practice of pharmacy." The FDA cautions, however, that the presence of a third party in the distribution of a prescription drug, between the nuclear pharmacy where the product is formulated, compounded, or manufactured from FDA-approved reagents and the point where it is administered to the patients, changes the practice to one of manufacturing.

18.5 STATE AND LOCAL REGULATORY AGENCIES

Other regulatory agencies include state-level agencies responsible for professional licensure of physicians, pharmacists, and technologists. Currently, only a few states have specialty licensure programs for nuclear medicine technologists. Several state boards of pharmacy require licensure for nuclear pharmacists, and many others are considering adoption of regulations to cover this specialty practice area. Such nuclear pharmacy regulations, however, are not intended to limit the preparation and dispensing of radiopharmaceuticals to pharmacists only. Generally, these regulations are concerned with nuclear pharmacy as practiced by commercial centralized nuclear pharmacies.

18.6 DEPARTMENT OF TRANSPORTATION

The Department of Transportation (DOT) is the primary federal agency that controls the interstate transport of hazardous substances, including radioactive materials. Specifically, DOT regulates the mode by which these materials may be transported (the NRC requires that transportation of radiopharmaceuticals between licensed users and manufacturers or suppliers meet DOT regulations).

Very simply, DOT regulations permit the transportation of radioactive materials so long as there is adequate containment of these materials and the radiation emitted by them. The packaging classification for radioactive materials is as follows:

Type A—Packaging is adequate to prevent loss or dispersal of a limited amount of radioactive material and to maintain proper radiation shielding during normal transport conditions.

Type B—Packaging is designed to safely contain very large quantities of radioactivity. Type B packaging is considerably more accident-resistant than Type A packaging.

Most radiopharmaceuticals are shipped in Type A packaging. Packages containing radioactive materials must be labeled ac-

Table 18–6.   Labeling classifications for packages containing radioactive materials.

Class	Special Handling*	Dose Rate (mR/hr)	
		Surface	At 1 m
Category I (white)	No	0.5	—
Category II (yellow)	Yes	50	1.0
Category III (yellow)	Yes†	200	10

*Special handling requirements include segregation from other packages.
†Vehicles which carry Category III (yellow) labeled packages must be placarded "Radioactive."

cording to one of three categories* (Table 18–6).

All three label types contain the distinctive trefoil symbol (Fig. 18–1), with one, two, or three bright red bars on either a white background only (one bar) or white and yellow background (two and three bars).

When required, packages must bear two identifying warning labels affixed to opposite sides of the outer package. Package labels must specify the contents (radionuclide) and amount of radioactivity (in either curies, millicuries, or microcuries); units must be marked either "Type A" or "Type B" in letters at least one-half inch high.

While DOT regulates the packaging and transportation of radioactive materials, individual pilots of commercial aircraft decide *when* these approved materials may be flown on passenger-carrying aircraft. Most radiopharmaceuticals (particularly those containing short-lived radionuclides) are shipped on regularly scheduled passenger-carrying aircraft because of the greater numbers of available flights and usually dependable time schedules. Based upon an agreement with the Airlines Pilots Association (ALPA), airlines permit pilots to review their freight cargo manifest and to

---

*Certain small quantities of radioactive materials are exempt from specified packaging and labeling requirements provided that (1) radiation reading at any external point on the package is less than 0.5 mrem/hr, (2) the materials are packaged to prevent leaks, and (3) the exterior of the package has no significant removable contamination. (The outside of the inner container must still bear the marking "Radioactive.")

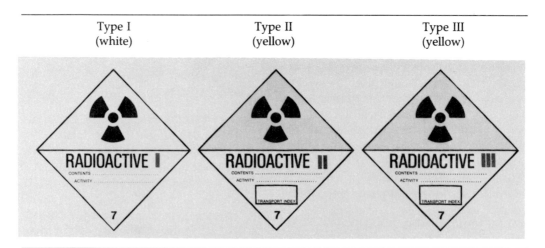

Type I (white)   Type II (yellow)   Type III (yellow)

The one-bar label has white background, while the two- and three-bar labels have bright yellow backgrounds on the upper halves of the label and white lower halves.

Fig. 18–1.   The label types for packages containing radioactive materials.

refuse those materials that they feel might endanger passenger safety. For this reason, shipments of radiopharmaceuticals are occasionally "bumped" by pilots from scheduled flights. This unfortunate decision often delays needed diagnostic or therapeutic procedures involving these radiopharmaceuticals.

Listed below are Active Regulatory Guides of the Nuclear Regulatory Commission which are available upon request (Write: Publications Service Section, Division of Technical Information and Document Control, United States Nuclear Regulatory Commission, Washington, D.C. 20555).

Guide 10.2 (Revision 1) Guidance to Academic Institutions Applying for Specific Byproduct Material Licenses of Limited Scope (1976)

Guide 10.5 (Revision 1) Applications for Type A Licenses of Broad Scope (1980)

Guide 10.8 (Revision 1) Guide for the Preparation of Applications for Medical Programs (1980)

REFERENCES

1. Code of Federal Regulations, Title 10 Energy, parts 0–199, US Government Printing Office, Washington, D.C., 1983.
2. Code of Federal Regulations, Title 49 Transportation, Parts 170–189, US Government Printing Office, Washington, D.C., 1983.
3. HEW, FDA. Guidelines for the clinical evaluation of radiopharmaceutical drugs: 77–3044. Superintendent of Documents, Washington, 1977.
4. Nuclear Pharmacy Guideline: Criteria for Determining When to Register as a Drug Establishment. Published by Division of Drug Labeling Compliance, Office of Compliance (HEN–310) Center for Drugs and Biologics. Rockville, MD, FDA. May 1984.
5. Swanson, DP, Lieto, RP: The submission of IND applications for radiopharmaceutical research: when and why. J Nucl Med 25:714–719, 1984.
6. US Department of Transportation. A review of the department of transportation (DOT). Regulations for transportation of radioactive materials. Research and Special Programs Administration, Materials Transportation Bureau, Washington, D.C., 1983.

Radiation Control and Protection

In nuclear pharmacy and nuclear medicine, radiation exposure is a routine component of the working environment. In the nuclear pharmacy, personnel exposure occurs not only during the preparation and dispensing of radiopharmaceuticals but also through contamination of the working environment wherever large sources of radioactivity (such as the ^{99}Mo-^{99m}Tc generator) are used. Exposure of personnel also occurs from radiopharmaceutical administration and from patients who have received these agents.

To reduce the radiation exposure of personnel to safe levels, several actions can be taken that collectively involve the implementation of a radiation protection plan. This plan requires the establishment of rules and regulations covering the handling, use, and disposal of radionuclides to restrict unnecessary exposure to radioactive materials along the ALARA concept (Section 18–3).

19.1 METHODS FOR REDUCING RADIATION EXPOSURE

The principal methods of reducing radiation exposure from external sources involve three basic elements—*time, distance,* and *shielding.*

Time. Since radiation dose is directly proportional to the length of exposure, time spent near radioactivity should be minimized.

Distance. Radiation dose-rate (the dose per time) from any external point source varies inversely as the square of the distance from the source. For instance, the dose-rate, R, at any distance, d, from a point source compared to the rate at a given distance, R_0, can be determined by the following mathematical expression.

$$R = \frac{R_0}{d^2}$$

Thus, at a point twice the distance from a radioactive source, the radiation exposure is reduced to one-fourth (i.e., $\frac{1}{2^2}$) the original rate. For this reason, it is desirable whenever practical to use forceps or tongs instead of picking up large amounts of radioactivity directly with the hands.

Shielding. Gamma radiation can be effectively shielded by using lead containers or bricks. The thickness of shielding material is usually given as the half-value layer (HVL), which is the amount of material (usually lead) required to reduce the dose-rate to one half its original value (Table 19–1). Each successive HVL reduces the transmitted radiation by about one half.

Lead-shielded syringe holders and leaded glass viewing windows in dose-drawing stations are beneficial in reducing exposure. While the use of syringe shields (Fig. 19–1) may initially appear awkward and time-consuming, studies have shown that hand, finger, and total body exposures during radiopharmaceutical preparation and administration can be reduced by as much as 50 to 80% when syringe shields are used.

ALARA policy is being implemented by

Table 19–1. Half-value layer (HVL) in lead (Pb) for selected radionuclides.

Radionuclide	Primary Photon Energy (KeV)	HVL (mm Pb)
I-125	27.5	0.04
Tc-99m	140	0.27
I-131	364	3.0
C-11, N-13, O-15, F-18	511	4.1
Cr-51	320	2.0
Fe-59	1095, 1292	11.0
Co-57	122, 136	3.0
Cs-137	662	6.5
Se-75	136, 265, 280	2.0

the NRC, especially in the areas of syringe shield use and release of radioactive materials to the environment. Radioactive materials licensees are now required to use syringe and vial shields to the maximum degree possible.

19.2 HANDLING AND RECEIPT OF RADIOACTIVE MATERIALS

When shipments of radioactive materials are received, it may be necessary to check packages for the presence of removable

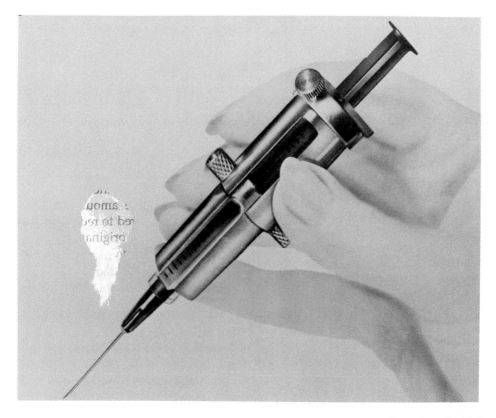

Fig. 19–1. Syringe shields are available to accommodate almost any size syringe. The syringe shield shown has a small window of leaded glass for viewing syringe contents during dose preparation and injection. (Courtesy Atomic Products Corporation.)

Table 19–2. Selected radionuclides and activities which do not necessarily require wipe-testing upon receipt (10 CFR Part 20.205b).

Radionuclide*	Wipe-testing not required if package contains less than (mCi)
Co-57	1
Co-57 (capsule)	20,000
Ga-67	100
In-111	100
I-123	100
I-125	10
I-131	100
I-131 (capsule)	3,000
Fe-59	1
Mo-99 (generator)	20,000
P-32	100
Se-75	1
Tc-99m	100
Tl-201	100
Yb-169	1
Xe-133 (saline)	100
Cr-51	100

*In liquid form unless otherwise noted.

contamination. Specifically, NRC regulations (and those of most Agreement States) require that licensees receiving certain packages of radioactive materials monitor for surface contamination within specified time limits. Some packages of radioactive materials are exempt from these surveys (Table 19–2); however, regulatory agencies require all licensees to have procedures for safely opening packages of radioactive materials, and some licensees elect to monitor (or wipe-test) all packages as a part of their package-opening procedure.

The *wipe-test* for the presence of radioactivity is accomplished by wiping the package surface (over an area approximately 100 cm²) with an absorbent paper, then counting it in an appropriate radiation detector. If removable radioactive contamination on the package surface exceeds 0.01 μCi (22,000 disintegrations per minute) per 100 cm², the licensee is required to immediately notify the final delivering carrier and the NRC (or Agreement State Agency) as well as any local licensing agency. Packages should be wipe-tested as soon as possible, but not later than 3 hours after receipt if received during normal working hours,

or 18 hours if received during off-duty hours. (See Appendix E.)

19.3 REDUCING EXPOSURE FROM INTERNAL RADIONUCLIDES

The handling of unsealed radioactive sources can result in internal contamination either by ingestion or inhalation (penetration through the skin is usually not a major avenue of entry).

Ingestion of uncontrolled radionuclides is probably the most important source of internal contamination (from spillage during transfer of radioactivity, patient excreta and sweat, contaminated linens, etc.). The major rules to minimize this problem are basic "good-housekeeping" guidelines and include the following:

1. Do not eat, drink, smoke, apply cosmetics, or pipette by mouth in areas in which radionuclides are used.
2. Wear protective gloves and lab coats when handling radioactivity.
3. Perform work involving radioactive materials on absorbent paper.
4. Exercise care when handling sheets and pillows that may be contami-

nated from patient sweat, blood, saliva, or urine.

5. Do not store food and drinks in the same area (i.e., refrigerator) as radioactive materials.

Inhalation is most likely to occur when handling gases such as radioactive xenon or volatile radionuclides such as I-131. In areas where these radionuclides are used it is desirable to have a slight negative air pressure with return ventilation separated from other systems in order to prevent the spread of radioactivity to other areas of the hospital. In addition, fume-type atmospheric exhaust hood should be used while storing or handling radioactive gases and volatile radionuclides, and a gas-trapping system should be used to collect radioactive gases after use in the patient.

Laboratory Surveys

The NRC requires that adequate surveys be performed to monitor laboratories (i.e., nuclear pharmacies) for external exposure to personnel, for surface contamination levels, and (when appropriate) for concentrations of airborne radioactive materials in the environment. These surveys, which are considered part of a comprehensive radiation protection program consistent with the ALARA philosophy, should include any location where individuals may be exposed to radiation intensities that might cause the occupational dose to exceed 10% of the MPD limits in any calendar quarter or where any radiation source could produce radiation levels greater than 1.0 mR/hr at a distance of one meter. Results of these surveys should be recorded. (See Appendix F.)

Sealed Sources

The NRC requires that all sealed sources of radioactivity, such as reference standards used in instrument calibration and quality control checks, be checked for con-

tamination or leakage at least twice a year. This is usually accomplished by wipe-testing the surface of the sealed source.

19.4 MAXIMUM PERMISSIBLE CONCENTRATION (MPC)

Radioactive gases such as radioxenon (Xe-133 and Xe-127) and volatile solutions of I-131 have the potential to leak into the atmosphere. Maximum permissible concentrations (MPC) for Xe-133 and I-131 (taken from 10 CFR Part 20) for air in occupational (restricted) and unrestricted areas are listed in Table 19–3.

In restricted areas exposure is assumed to be 40 hours/week, while in unrestricted areas longer occupancy is assumed. MPC values in unrestricted areas may be averaged over a one-year period, allowing higher radionuclide levels over short periods as long as the yearly average is less than the concentrations (MPC values). Adherence to the ALARA concepts, however, dictates that concentration values be maintained as low as possible.

19.5 HANDLING VOLATILE AND GASEOUS RADIONUCLIDES

Atmospheric exhaust hoods are used in nuclear medicine for handling and storing volatile radionuclides that might cause airborne contamination. These hoods are very much like those used in chemical laboratories to exhaust hazardous fumes directly to the atmosphere. Atmospheric exhaust hoods are not usually considered to be a method of disposal for radioactive materials because stringent regulations govern the types and amounts of radionuclides that can be released to the atmosphere. Some atmospheric exhaust hoods built for nuclear medicine facilities have special filters that trap radionuclides to prevent their release into the atmosphere. The minimum average face velocity of air in a fume hood should not be less than 100 linear feet/minute. Additionally, the exhaust outlet should be at a point 5 to 10 feet above the

Table 19–3. Maximum permissible concentrations in air* for I-131 and Xe-133.

Radionuclide	MPC in air, μCi/cm³	
	Restricted Area	Unrestricted Area
I-131	9×10^{-9}	1×10^{-10}
Xe-133	1×10^{-5}	3×10^{-7}

*10 CFR Part 20

roof of the building and at a minimum of 25 feet from the nearest heating, air conditioning, or other intake mechanism to prevent re-entry of contamination into the building.

While exhaust hoods are effective in protecting personnel from gaseous types of radioactive contamination, these hoods are usually not designed to provide a sterile environment. When a sterile working environment is necessary for the preparation of pharmaceuticals, the use of a laminar-flow hood is required. Laminar-flow hoods prevent airborne bacterial contamination from reaching the work area; however, volatile forms of radioactivity may be picked up by the clean air stream and distributed into the environment.

19.6 BIOASSAY FOR RADIOIODIDE

As described in Regulatory Guide 8.20, routine bioassays should be considered when individuals handle unsealed quantities of volatile I-125 and I-131 that exceed those levels shown in Table 19–4. The quantities apply to single events or to the total amount of radioactivity handled by an individual in a three-month period.

Bioassay for radioiodine is usually facilitated in nuclear medicine laboratories by the presence of equipment routinely used to measure thyroid uptake of I-131 in patients (bioassay for radioxenons is not required since these radionuclides are physiologically inert).

19.7 DISPOSAL OF RADIOACTIVE WASTES

In nuclear medicine, radioactive waste materials (contaminated patient injection paraphernalia such as syringes, needles, etc. and residual amounts of radioactivity in vials) may be disposed of by several methods. These include:

1. Storage of material for decay
2. Burial in soil (with special permission)
3. Release into a sanitary sewer system
4. Transfer to authorized recipient (commercial waste sites)
5. Other approved disposal methods (including incineration and atmospheric release of radioactive gases).

Storage of Materials for Decay.   Radiopharmaceuticals that contain short-lived radionuclides, such as Tc-99m, may be stored for sufficient periods (usually ten half-lives) until the amount of radioactivity is not detectable above background levels, then disposed of as regular trash. A low level survey instrument set on its most sen-

Table 19–4. Levels of radioactivity for I-125 or I-131 above which bioassay is necessary (NRC Regulatory Guide 8.20).

Type of Operation	Volatile or Dispersible Form*
1. Open room or bench with possible escape from container	1 mCi
2. Possible escape, process in fume hood of adequate design and reliability	10 mCi
3. In glovebox	100 mCi

*When using I-131/I-125 bound as a nonvolatile agent (e.g., capsules), the activity levels are higher by a factor of 10.

sitive range is used to monitor for radioactivity (with all shielding removed) in a low-background area. Before disposal, all radioactive labels and warnings must be removed.

Burial in Soil. In the past, licensees of radioactive materials were permitted by the NRC (or the appropriate state-level agency) to bury radioactive wastes in soil. The provisions for this disposal method were abolished a few years ago. Special permission is needed to continue this practice.

Release into a Sanitary Sewer System. NRC regulations permit disposal of radionuclides into sewage, with amounts determined by MPC values of radionuclides in water as given in 10 CFR Part 20. Disposal depends on the rate of flow of sewage water but is limited to 1 curie per year of *total* radioactivity, with the limits for C-14 and H-3 set at 1 and 5 curies, respectively, in addition to this total. (Radiopharmaceuticals excreted in urine or feces and passed into sanitary sewers are *not* considered as having been disposed of by this method.)

Transfer to Authorized Recipient. In order to dispose of very long-lived radionuclides it may be necessary to use commercial waste disposal facilities. These facilities are authorized to dispose of materials either by burial at approved sites or by incineration.

Other Approved Methods of Disposal. Depending on the physical form and volume of radioactive wastes, disposal methods other than those previously mentioned may be utilized. Incineration, with regulatory agency approval, is one method by which institutions may dispose of the carcasses of research animals that contain radioactive materials. In limited quantities, radioactive gases may be released into the atmosphere; most institutions, however, have developed ALARA programs for trapping expired Xenon-133 and Xenon-127 using specialized xenon-charcoal trapping devices. Several commercial systems

are available that use activated charcoal to trap xenon. These gas-trapping devices, with each repeated use, move xenon along the length of the charcoal trap in a stepwise fashion. Eventually (and with proper use), the radioactive xenon should decay before reaching the end of the charcoal trap and exiting with the trap effluent. It may be necessary, however, to replace these charcoal cartridges at periodic intervals, since continued use may result in saturated xenon binding capacity. Additionally, since moisture prevents xenon bindig to charcoal, desiccants should be used to "dry" the expired xenon before it is placed in the trap. These desiccants must also be replaced frequently. To ensure that no appreciable amounts of xenon are being released, several manufacturers of xenon traps have included detection devices at the outlet port to monitor xenon leakage. Gas-trapping systems (with or without built-in detection devices) should be checked routinely to ensure optimum trap performance.

19.8 BASIC RULES IN NUCLEAR PHARMACY AREAS

The following basic rules should be observed in the nuclear pharmacy when working with radioactive materials:

1. Lab coats and disposable gloves should be worn at all times.
2. All working surfaces and transport elements (carts, etc.) should be covered with absorbent paper that has a nonpermeable plastic coating on the reverse side.
3. Radioactive materials should be kept in closed, shielded containers at all times.
4. All shielded containers should bear a label identifying the radiopharmaceutical, the amounts of radioactivity, and the date of assay.
5. All spills should be cleaned immediately.
6. Eating, drinking, smoking, and ap-

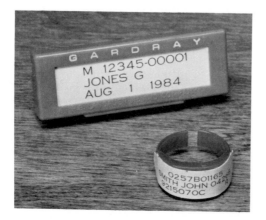

Fig. 19–2. Example of types of film badges (standard badge and ring badge) used for routine personnel monitoring. (Courtesy R.S. Landauer, Jr. and Company.)

plication of cosmetics should be prohibited in areas where radioactive materials are stored or handled.

7. Personnel film badges should be worn at all times when handling materials or working in those areas where radioactive materials are handled or stored.
8. Food and drinks should not be stored in the same area as radioactive materials.

19.9   PERSONNEL MONITORING

There are three major types of devices used to measure the radiation dose to laboratory personnel. They are the film badge, the thermoluminescent dosimeter (TLD), and the pocket ionization chamber.

Film Badges. As the name implies, these devices rely on the blackening of sensitive film in order to estimate radiation dose. Filters (aluminum, copper, tin, or lead) are used in the film badge (Fig. 19–2) to differentiate radiations of different types and energies. Film badges, which are the most widely used personnel dosimeters, are usually collected monthly for film development and reading.

TLD Badges. These devices usually use small chips of lithium fluoride held in hold-

ers similar to film badges. When the chips absorb radiation, alterations in electron configuration occur within the crystal, with the electrons absorbing energy and being raised to excited energy levels. Subsequent heating causes the electrons to return to their normal state, and the material gives off measurable amounts of light that are proportional to the radiation dose.

Pocket Ionization Dosimeters. These ionization devices, described in Chapter 4, allow an immediate determination of radiation exposure, either by reading the dosimeter directly or by placing the dosimeter in a charger/reader device. Pocket ionization dosimeters are most helpful when handling large amounts of radioactivity.

19.10   RADIATION AREAS AND POSTING

Radiation Areas

NRC regulations designate two specific types of "areas," restricted and unrestricted, prescribed by different radiation limits. In a *restricted area* access is controlled by the licensee to assure protection from radiation and radioactive materials. Normally, restricted areas include departmental areas occupied by individuals employed to work with radioactive materials and are not accessible to the general public. *Unrestricted areas* are readily accessible to the general public. The permissible radiation in these areas is as follows:

- *Unrestricted areas* are those areas in which a person continuously present would receive a dose exceeding neither 2 mrem in any 1 hour nor 100 mrem in any 7 consecutive days.
- *Restricted areas* would exceed the levels for unrestricted areas and would require control of access.

Posting

The NRC requires that specific signs be used to warn of possible danger from the

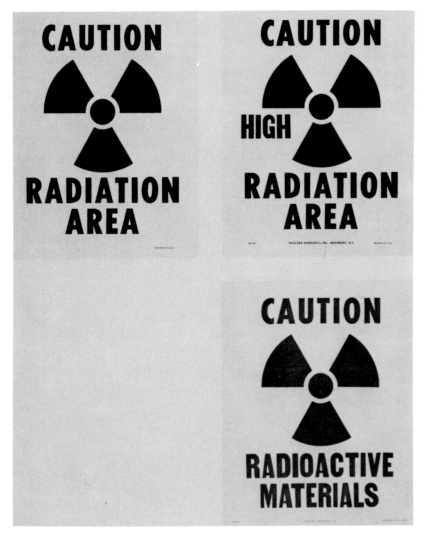

Fig. 19–3. Signs required by the NRC to warn of possible danger from the presence of either radioactive materials or radiation.

presence of radiation. These signs use magenta or purple colors on a yellow background and incorporate the conventional trefoil radiation symbol (Fig. 19–3).

1. *Caution: Radiation Area.* Signs with these words and the radiation symbol are used to designate areas in which there is the possibility of a dose of greater than 5 mrem in an hour to a major body part or more than 100 mrem in 5 consecutive days.

2. *Caution: High Radiation Area.* These signs designate areas in which an individual might receive to a major body part a dose in excess of 100 mrem in an hour. Such areas require warning signals or controls that may include visible or audible alarm signals.

3. *Caution: Radioactive Materials.* In general, *rooms* in which radioactive materials are used or stored must be posted with this warning. This label is also required on *containers* in which quantities of radioactive material are stored or used (additionally, labeling

should always include the radionuclide, the amount of activity present, and the date of assay).

4. *Caution: Airborne Radioactivity Area.* This sign is required if airborne activity exceeds at any time the MPC in air for 40 hours of occupational exposure (see Table 19–3).

19.11 RADIOPHARMACEUTICAL MISADMINISTRATIONS

According to NRC (10 CFR Part 35), misadministration of a radiopharmaceutical is defined as the administration of a radiopharmaceutical other than the one intended, the administration of a radiopharmaceutical to the wrong patient, or the administration of a radiopharmaceutical by an administration route or in a quantity* other than that prescribed.

---

*An incorrect quantity differs from the prescribed quantity by more than 50% for diagnostic radiopharmaceuticals; incorrect therapeutic dosages differ by more than 10%.

REFERENCES

1. Barrall, RC, Smith, SI: Personnel radiation exposure and protection from ^{99m}Tc radiations. *In* AAPM Monograph No. 1, Biophysical Aspects of the Medical Use of Technetium-99m. Edited by JG Kereiakes, KR Corey. Cincinnati, American Association of Physicists in Medicine, 1976.
2. Bolmsjö, MS, Persson, BRR: Factors affecting the trapping performance of Xenon holdup-filters in nuclear medicine application. Med Phys 9:96–105, 1982.
3. Burr, JE, Berg, R: Radiation dose to hands from radiopharmaceuticals—preparation versus injection. J Nucl Med Tech 5:158–160, 1977.
4. Code of Federal Regulations, Title 10 Energy, Part 20, Washington, D.C., US Government Printing Office, 1983.
5. ICRP Publication 25. The Handling, Storage, Use and Disposal of Unsealed Radionuclides in Hospitals and Medical Research Establishments. New York, International Commission on Radiological Protection, Pergamon Press, 1976.
6. NCRP Report No. 39. Basic Radiation Protection Criteria. Washington, D.C., National Council on Radiation Protection and Measurements, 1971.

Appendix A

Exponential (E) table. To determine the fraction of radioactivity remaining (A) at time t, the equation $A = A_0 e^{-\lambda t}$ can be used where A_0 = original activity and $\lambda = 0.693/T\frac{1}{2}$. The exponential table can be used by allowing $\lambda t = x$, then locating the corresponding $e^{-\lambda t}$ value. The value obtained is employed as the decay factor.

x	e^{-x}	x	e^{-x}	x	e^{-x}
0.00	1.000	0.40	0.670	1.0	0.368
0.01	0.990	0.41	0.664	1.1	0.333
0.02	0.980	0.42	0.657	1.2	0.301
0.03	0.970	0.43	0.651	1.3	0.273
0.04	0.961	0.44	0.644	1.4	0.247
0.05	0.951	0.45	0.638	1.5	0.223
0.06	0.942	0.46	0.631	1.6	0.202
0.07	0.932	0.47	0.625	1.7	0.183
0.08	0.923	0.48	0.619	1.8	0.165
0.09	0.914	0.49	0.613	1.9	0.150
0.10	0.905	0.50	0.607	2.0	0.135
0.11	0.896	0.52	0.595	2.1	0.122
0.12	0.887	0.54	0.583	2.2	0.111
0.13	0.878	0.56	0.571	2.3	0.100
0.14	0.869	0.58	0.560	2.4	0.0907
0.15	0.861			2.5	0.0821
0.16	0.852	0.60	0.549	2.6	0.0743
0.17	0.844	0.62	0.538	2.7	0.0672
0.18	0.835	0.64	0.527	2.8	0.0608
0.19	0.827	0.66	0.517	2.9	0.0550
		0.68	0.507		
0.20	0.819			3.0	0.0498
0.21	0.811	0.70	0.497	3.2	0.0408
0.22	0.803	0.72	0.487	3.4	0.0334
0.23	0.795	0.74	0.477	3.6	0.0273
0.24	0.787	0.76	0.468	3.8	0.0224
0.25	0.779	0.78	0.458		
0.26	0.771			4.0	0.0183
0.27	0.763	0.80	0.449	4.2	0.0150
0.28	0.756	0.82	0.440	4.4	0.0123
0.29	0.748	0.84	0.432	4.6	0.0101
		0.86	0.423	4.8	0.0082
		0.88	0.415		
0.30	0.741				
0.31	0.733			5.0	0.0067
0.32	0.726	0.90	0.407	5.5	0.0041
0.33	0.719	0.92	0.399	6.0	0.0025
0.34	0.712	0.94	0.391	6.5	0.0015
0.35	0.705	0.96	0.383	7.0	0.0009
0.36	0.698	0.98	0.375	7.5	0.0006
0.37	0.691			8.0	0.0003
0.38	0.684			8.5	0.0002
0.39	0.677			9.0	0.0001

Appendix B

Radiation absorbed dose (mrad/μCi) from specific radioactive agents commonly used in patients (NCRP–70).

Radio-pharmaceutical Agent	Mode of Administration	Physical Half-Life	Source Organ	Biological Assumptions Fraction Administered Activity	Biological Half-Time	Radiation Absorbed Dose (in adults) Tissue	mrad/μCi
P-32 phosphate	IV	14.3 days	Liver	0.02	49 days	Liver	6.3
			Spleen	0.02	49 days	Spleen	63
			Skeleton	0.63	49 days	Total bone	56
			Rest of body	0.33	49 days	Testes	3
						Red marrow	57
						Total body	8.1
Cr-51 red blood cells	IV	27.7 days	Blood			Blood	0.31
			Spleen			Ovaries	0.29
						Red marrow	0.31
						Spleen	14
						Testes	0.23
						Total body	0.31
Fe-59 chloride	IV	45 days	Kidney	0.0293	800 days	Kidneys	84
			Liver	0.2227	800 days	Liver	120
			Lungs	0.0206	800 days	Lungs	34
			Spleen	0.0369	800 days	Spleen	150
			Testes	0.0094	800 days	Ovaries	20
			Rest of body	0.6811	800 days	Testes	150
						Red marrow	21
						Total body	23
Co-57 vitamin B$_{12}$	Oral	270 days	Liver	0.46	91.3 days	Liver	110
			Stomach	0.02	91.3 days	Stomach wall	17
			Spleen	0.0035	91.3 days	Spleen	10
			Kidneys	0.0144	91.3 days	Kidneys	25
			Ovaries	0.00018	91.3 days	Total bone	3.5
			Bone	0.01	91.3 days	Ovaries	5.7
			Testes	0.0076	91.3 days	Testes	61
			Rest of body	0.0038	91.3 days	Red marrow	4.5
						Total body	5.8
Ga-67 citrate	IV	78.0 hr			30hr 613hr	GI Tract	
			Spleen	0.0072	17% 83%	Stomach	0.22
			Kidneys	0.0076	17% 83%	S.I.	0.36
			Adrenals	0.0006	17% 83%	U.L.I.	0.56
			Marrow	0.054	17% 83%	L.L.I.	0.90
			Liver	0.050	17% 83%	Ovaries	0.28
			Bone	0.18	17% 83%		

Radiopharmaceutical	Route	$T_{1/2}$	Source organ	Fraction	Effective half-time	Target organ	Dose
Kr-81m gas	Inhalation and Rebreathing	13 sec	Lung	0.95	0.35 min	Liver	0.012
			Rest of body	0.05	5 min	Lungs	.0002
						Red marrow	.00013
						Ovaries	1.8×10^{-5}
						Spleen	.00019
						Testes	5.9×10^{-5}
						Total body	.00029
Tc-99m pentetate (DTPA)	IV	6 hr	Kidney	0.90	5.95 hr	Bladder wall	0.28
			Rest of body	0.10	5.95 hr	Kidneys	0.74
			Bladder contents			Ovaries	0.013
						Testes	0.0057
						Red marrow	0.018
						Total body	0.011
Tc-99m albumin macroaggre-gates	IV	6 hr	Liver	0.015	250 hr	Bladder wall	0.29
				0.045	9 hr	Liver	0.030
				0.090	0.5 hr	Lungs	0.21
			Lung	0.80	7.8 hr	Ovaries	0.0085
			Rest of body	0.05	∞	Testes	0.0052
			Bladder contents			Red marrow	0.011
						Total body	0.012
Tc-99m microspheres (15 to 22 μm)	IV	6 hr	Lung	0.57	45 hr	Bladder wall	0.17
			Rest of body	0.37	4 hr	Ovaries	0.0060
			Bladder contents	0.06	∞	Testes	0.0036
						Red marrow	0.013
						Lung	0.26
						Total body	0.014
Tc-99m diphosphonate	IV	6 hr	Bladder contents	0.5	∞	Bladder wall	0.051
			Bone	0.1	∞	Total bone	0.051
			Rest of body	0.4	0.5 hr	Red marrow	0.033
						Ovaries	0.0080
						Testes	0.0061
						Total body	0.012
Tc-99m disofenin	IV	6 hr	Liver			U.L.I.	0.55
			Large intestine			Liver	0.09
						Red marrow	0.02
						Ovaries	0.05
						Testes	0.03
Tc-99m gluceptate	IV	6 hr	Kidney			Kidney	0.30
						Red marrow	0.012
						Gonads	0.005
						Total body	0.01

Radiopharmaceutical Agent	Mode of Administration	Physical Half-Life	Source Organ	Fraction Administered Activity	Biological Half-Time	Tissue	mrad/μCi a	mrad/μCi b
Tc-99m DMSA (succimer)	IV	6 hr	Kidney	0.60		Renal cortex	1.40	
			Total body	0.33		Red marrow	0.02	
			Liver	0.05		Gonads	0.02	
Tc-99m red blood cells	IV	6 hr	Total body	1	∞	Liver	0.019	
						Red marrow	0.025	
						Spleen	0.019	
						Ovaries	0.021	
						Testes	0.014	
						Total body	0.017	
Tc-99m sodium pertechnetate	IV	6 hr	Extra-vascular	a—resting population		Bladder wall	0.053	0.085
			Large intestine	b—nonresting population		Stomach (wall)	0.25	0.051
			Plasma			Upper large int. (wall)	0.068	0.12
			Red blood cells			Lower large int. (wall)	0.061	0.11
			Salivary glands			Ovaries	0.022	0.030
			Stomach			Red marrow	0.019	0.017
			Thyroid			Testes	0.009	0.009
						Thyroid	0.13	0.13
						Total body	0.014	0.011
Tc-99m sulfur colloid	IV	6 hr	Liver	0.85	∞	Liver	0.34	
			Spleen	0.07	∞	Ovaries	0.0056	
			Red marrow	0.05	∞	Red marrow	0.027	
			Rest of body	0.03	∞	Spleen	0.21	
						Testes	0.0011	
						Total body	0.019	
In-111 chloride	IV	2.83 days	Liver	0.33	∞	Liver	4.5	
			Red marrow	0.33	∞	Red marrow	2.8	
			Rest of body	0.33	∞	Spleen	0.41	
						Ovaries	0.52	
						Testes	0.21	
						Total body	0.6	

Biological Assumptions (Fraction Administered Activity, Biological Half-Time); Radiation Absorbed Dose (in adults) (Tissue, mrad/μCi)

Radiopharmaceutical	Route	Physical half-life	Source organs	Notes	Timing	Target organ	Dose
I-123 sodium iodide	Oral	13 hr	Intestine, Liver, Stomach, Thyroid	Maximum thyroid uptake of 15%		Liver	0.028
						Ovaries	0.034
						Red marrow	0.030
						Stomach wall	0.23
						Testes	0.012
						Thyroid	7.5
						Total body	0.027
I-123 sodium rose bengal	IV	13 hr	Liver and biliary tract		0.67 hr	Gall bladder wall	0.25
			Contents of gall bladder			GI tract small intestine	0.60
			Small intestine and contents		0.36 hr	Upper large int. (wall)	1
			Contents of upper large intestine		0.11 hr	Lower large int. (wall)	1.5
			Contents of lower large intestine		0.06 hr	Liver	0.19
						Ovaries	0.28
						Red marrow	0.080
						Testes	0.014
I-125 sodium iodide	Oral	60.2 days	Intestine, Liver, Stomach, Thyroid	Maximum thyroid uptake of 15%		Liver	0.22
						Ovaries	0.033
						Red marrow	0.077
						Stomach wall	0.26
						Testes	0.018
						Thyroid	450.
						Total body	0.29
I-131 sodium iodide	Oral	8.06 days	Intestine, Liver, Stomach, Thyroid	Maximum thyroid uptake of 15%		Liver	0.35
						Ovaries	0.14
						Red marrow	0.20
						Stomach wall	1.6
						Testes	0.085
						Thyroid	800.
						Total body	0.47
I-131 orthoiodo-hippuric acid	IV	8.06 days	Total body	0.0125	7.5 hr	Bladder wall	13.
				0.085	1 hr	Kidneys	0.41
				0.4025	0.3 hr	Ovaries	0.073
			Kidney	0.01	12 hr	Testes	0.053
				0.05	50 min	Red marrow	0.021
				0.10	10 min	Total body	0.028
				0.34	2 min		

Radio-pharmaceutical Agent	Mode of Administration	Physical Half-Life	Source Organ	Biological Assumptions		Radiation Absorbed Dose (in adults)	
				Fraction Administered Activity	Biological Half-Time	Tissue	mrad/μCi
Xe-127 gas	Ventilation	36.4 days	Spirometer volume of 5 liters			Lungs	0.0047
						Red marrow	0.0017
						Ovaries	0.0014
						Testes	0.0010
						Total body	0.0013
Xe-133 gas	Ventilation	5.31 days	Spirometer volume of 5 liters			Lungs	0.011
						Red marrow	0.0015
						Ovaries	0.0013
						Testes	0.0012
						Total body	0.0014
Yb-169 DTPA	Intrathecal	32 days				Blood	0.10
						Spinal cord	13–49
						mean value	31
						Nerve roots	26–66
						mean value	46
						Brain	70
Tl-201 chloride	IV	73.1 hr	Stomach	0.0056	240 hr	GI tract	
			S.I.	0.0308	240 hr	Stomach wall	0.40
			U.L.I.	0.0024	240 hr	S.I.	0.38
			L.L.I.	0.0019	240 hr	U.L.I. wall	0.25
			Heart	0.038	27.8 hr	L.L.I. wall	0.21
			Kidneys	0.035	240 hr	Heart wall	0.50
			Liver	0.087	240 hr	Kidneys	1.2
			Ovaries	0.003		Liver	0.57
			Testes	0.0016	240 hr	Ovaries	0.47
			Thyroid	0.0015	240 hr	Testes	0.52
			Rest of body	0.7959		Thyroid	0.64
						Total body	0.21

Appendix C

Radiation exposure rates for selected radionuclides used in medicine and pharmacy.

Radionuclide	R/mCi/hr/cm	mr/hr for 1 mCi at 1 foot
Au-198	2.3	2.46
Co-60	12.8	13.7
Cs-137	3.26	3.48
Ga-67	1.6	1.71
In-111	3.2	3.42
I-123	2.2	2.35
I-131	2.2	2.35
Tc-99m	0.72	0.77
Tl-201	4.7	5.02
Xe-127	2.2	2.35
Xe-133	0.73	0.78

Appendix D

Absorbed dose to critical organs for selected radiopharmaceuticals in pediatric patients and adults.

Radionuclide	Chemical Form	Critical Organ	Critical Organ Dose (mrad/μCi administered)					
			Newborn	1 yr	5 yr	10 yr	15 yr	Adult
99mTc	pentetate (DTPA)	bladder[a]	5.00	1.70	1.10	0.80	0.56	0.45
		kidney	0.39	0.15	0.10	0.07	0.05	0.04
	disofenin	liver	0.79	0.37	0.25	0.15	0.11	0.09
	HSA	blood	0.81	0.24	0.15	0.09	0.06	0.05
	MAA (microspheres)	lung	3.09	1.00	0.59	0.35	0.26	0.20
	sodium pertechnetate	LLI[b]	1.91	0.67	0.46	0.33	0.23	0.20
	sulfur colloid	liver	2.90	1.34	0.92	0.56	0.40	0.33
123I	sodium iodide	thyroid	0.16	0.08	0.04	0.02	0.02	0.01
131I	sodium iodide	thyroid	16.0	8.09	3.78	2.22	1.55	1.11
99mTc	sodium pertechnetate	thyroid[c]	0.005	0.002	0.001	0.0006	0.0005	0.0003

[a] Assumes 6-hour bladder residence time.
[b] Perchlorate blocking dose (IV administration).
[c] Thyroid is not the critical organ for 99mTc-sodium pertechnetate; doses given for comparison to radioiodines.

From: NCRP No. 73

Appendix E

PROCEDURES FOR SAFELY OPENING PACKAGES CONTAINING RADIOACTIVE MATERIALS

1. Visually inspect package for any signs of damage (such as wetness or torn packing container).

2. Measure exposure rates at package surface and at three feet. If exposure rates are more than 200 or 10 mR/hr, respectively, discontinue check-in procedure immediately and notify institution's Radiation Safety personnel.

3. After putting on disposable gloves, open package outer container and remove packing slip. Open inner package to verify content (correct as shipped) and check integrity of final source container (inspect for breakage of seals or vials, loss of liquid, or discoloration of packaging materials). Check also that receipt of shipment does not exceed possession limits.

4. Wipe external surface of final source container with either moistened cotton swab or filter paper held with forceps; assay and record results.

5. Monitor the packing material and packages for contamination before discarding. *Note:* If contaminated, treat as radioactive waste. Otherwise, destroy all "radioactive" labeling on package and discard in regular trash.

In all the above procedures, take wipe-tests with appropriate absorbent material and with appropriate precaution against the spread of contamination, if present. Measurement should be made with a suitable detection instrument such as a thin-end-window GM survey meter or a multichannel analyzer (MCA) with a sodium-iodide (Tl) detector.

Appendix F

AREA SURVEY PROCEDURES

1. *Frequency*

   All generator elution, radiopharmaceutical preparation, and injection areas should be surveyed daily with a low-range thin-window GM survey meter and decontaminated,* if necessary. *Note*—laboratory areas where only small quantities of radioactive materials are used (less than 100 μCi) should be surveyed monthly. All other laboratory areas can be surveyed weekly.

2. *Survey Techniques*

   The weekly and monthly survey consist of:

   a. measurement of radiation levels with a survey meter sufficiently sensitive to detect 0.1 mRem/hr.

   b. a series of wipe-tests to measure contamination levels. This method should be sufficiently sensitive to detect 100 dpm cm^2 for the suspected radiocontaminant.

3. *Record Keeping*

   A permanent record will be kept of all survey results, including negative results. The record will include:

   a. location, date, and type of equipment used.

   b. name of person conducting survey.

   c. drawing of area surveyed, identifying relevant features such as storage and waste areas.

   d. measured exposure rates, keyed to location on area drawing (areas with high exposure rates that require corrective action should be identified).

   e. detected contamination levels, keyed to location on drawing.

   f. corrective action taken in case of contamination or excessive exposure rates, reduced contamination levels or exposure rates after corrective action, and any appropriate comments.

   For daily surveys where no abnormal exposures are found, only the date, the identification of the person performing the study, and the survey reports will be recorded.

---

*Areas will be cleaned if the contamination levels exceed 100 dpm/100 cm^2.

Index

Page numbers in *italics* indicate figures; numbers followed by "t" indicate tables; numbers followed by "n" indicate footnotes